REFLEX ZONE MASSAGE

Clearly and simply explains the principles and application
of reflexology of the feet and hands to facilitate the
effective use of this holistic treatment.

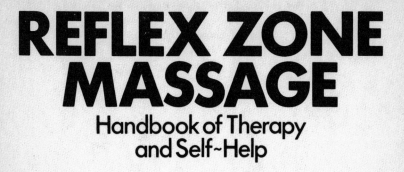

REFLEX ZONE MASSAGE

Handbook of Therapy and Self-Help

by

Franz Wagner Ph.D.

Foreword by Gaston St Pierre

Illustrated by Horst Linhart
Atelier Auberg, Linz

Translated from the German by
Linda Sonntag

THORSONS PUBLISHING GROUP

First published in the United Kingdom 1987

First published in Austria as *Reflexzonen Massage*
© Veritas-Verlag, Linz 1984

© THORSONS PUBLISHING GROUP 1987

British Library Cataloguing in Publication Data

Wagner, Franz
Reflex zone massage: handbook of therapy
and self-help.
1. Reflexotherapy
I. Title   II. Schwarz, Hans
III. Reflexzonen Massage. *English*
615.8'22   RM723.R43

ISBN 0-7225-1385-2

*Published by Thorsons Publishers Limited,
Wellingborough, Northamptonshire, NN8 2RQ England.*

Printed in Great Britain by
Biddles Limited, Guildford, Surrey.

3   5   7   9   10   8   6   4

For Vera Lisa, who has let me share with her the secret of life.

My thanks are due to Hans Schwarz whose advice was most valuable.

Thirty spokes meet at a hub—
The space between them makes the wheel.
The potter makes pots out of clay—
The emptiness inside makes the pot.

Doors and windows are breaks in walls—
The space inside them is the home.
Shapes are there for the eye to see
But their true value is invisible.

Laotse: *Tao-te-king XI*

Contents

Foreword

Throughout the ages it has seemed that, in the field of healing, energy was used as a therapeutic tool. This was in the form of potion, application, herbal pill, aspirin or homoeopathic tablet, or needle used by either the acupuncturist or doctor. Today, we are considering consciousness as a therapeutic tool. This new orientation was heralded in the works of Dr Sigmund Freud and of Dr Carl Gustav Jung. It has, over the last few decades, found a wider context of application aptly coined in the phrase *the holistic approach*.

In 1983, Franz Wagner and Hans Schwarz attended a seminar on Metamorphosis which I gave in Germany. I was struck by their enthusiastic response and intrigued at their readiness to discuss and appreciate the principles of my work, which concerns the development of consciousness during the gestation period, and the way in which the fluctuations in the flow of energy and consciousness *in utero* establish the patterns which control our lives now. After attending workshops where he learned and practised the Metamorphic Technique, Dr Wagner was instrumental in introducing Metamorphosis to Austria.

It is a mark of intelligence not only to make a success of one's chosen field but also to venture on to new ground and to go on being successful. From his own field of social science and university lecturing, Franz Wagner went on to explore the world of alternative medicine, more specifically, reflexology. Here, not satisfied with simply repeating what his predecessors had discovered and used over the centuries, he fully embraced the motion proposed by the 1982 Conference on Humanism in Salzburg: '*We don't need a new medical system—what we need is a new view of mankind!*' He applied his sense of sobriety, order and intelligence to consider 'the human nature of the human being' and thereby help man to help himself.

'*Holistic therapy sees man in terms of energy, healing powers and life forces. It is concerned with the forces flowing through the body which are the very essence of life itself. They determine personality and they determine physical characteristics, too . . .'*

Throughout his book, Franz Wagner goes on refining this definition while providing basic information on therapeutic training. The importance of the quality of the exchange between the therapist and the patient, and of the relationship between man and the world, is stressed. This relationship helps to stimulate the living forces, support the innate intelligence and activate the integration of all the healing factors within the person.

Dr Wagner reminds us that our trust in the natural methods of healing may give us more faith in ourselves and in life and that, above all, beyond sickness and health there is life.

I am glad that reflexology is finding in him such an innovative and creative presenter in this book which is accessible to all.

Gaston St Pierre
The Metamorphic Association,
London

Introduction

All kinds of different things may have prompted you to pick up this book, to buy it or decide to use it. It could be that you have heard about reflexology from a friend or are already acquainted with it yourself, in which case you might simply want to find out more about it. Or you could be working in the health services and have come across it that way. Perhaps you are unhappy that in the face of increasingly sophisticated equipment and technological advance in the sphere of medicine, the point of it all—the health and well-being of the individual, body and soul—has somehow got lost.

If you have acquired this book as part of a seminar or introductory course on the subject, then it will not be long before you will experience for yourself some of the potential of reflex zone massage. For a long time reflexology was regarded with scepticism and distrust. In more recent times, however, it has had such great success that it has ceased to be an outsider and has taken its place within the framework of holistic therapy, where it is gaining increasing respect and recognition from practitioners of conventional medicine.

It must be made quite clear at the outset that reflexology is not an alternative to orthodox medicine. Reflex zone therapy can play an important part in regulating the body's functions, but the greatest advantages are to be gained when therapist and doctor work together for the patient's health. Long experience has taught us how difficult it can sometimes be to find common ground between the two, and also how rewarding it is, once an understanding has been achieved.

The lack of communication between doctors and therapists is often due to the one-sided scientific approach of orthodox medicine, which can prevent doctors from seeking an all-round view of their patients. Diagnosis and therapy, though seemingly poles apart, do have points of contact and these should be made the most of. It should not be forgotten that reflexology (with other holistic treatments) and the traditional institutional-ized practices of orthodox medicine do after all share a common aim: to improve the health of their patients.

Reflex zone massage does not offer extensive opportunities for diagnosis—these remain the province of the doctor. What it does offer is an increasingly broad experience of the principles of holistic treatment. The technological advances continually being made in orthodox medicine often leave the doctor too little time for an intensive analysis of his patient's problems and needs, yet no one would deny the importance of the encounter between doctor and patient, which is a deeply human one that endeavours to break down barriers and establish a relationship of trust.

Reflexology is fundamentally concerned with the patient as an individual and its sometimes extraordinary success as a method of healing is based entirely on the relationship built up between the patient and his therapist. With these points in mind, it is to be hoped that therapists and doctors will find more opportunities for working alongside each other to their mutual advantage and for the good of their patients.

Reflexology can be a very effective method of treatment and of self-help, but its success does not depend merely on a topographical knowledge of the reflex zones on the feet and hands. The increasing interest in the techniques of reflexology is very encouraging, and the best way of learning is to get a thorough practical knowledge from a therapist during a course of demonstrations.

However, it must be said that not everyone who massages what he supposes to be the correct zones on the foot (and there are some misconceptions as to their identity) will get the hoped-for reaction in the corresponding part of the body. Certainly any massage treatment will increase the subject's well-being and stimulate the circulation. But a mistaken or misapplied treatment can also have unexpected consequences. (More of this in a later section.)

Much of what has been written and published about reflexology contains sweeping statements and broad generaliza-tions, and these lead the reader to believe that all he has to do is press the foot here and there to become a reflexologist. Our view of reflex zone massage of the feet is more specific: we see it as a holistic method of treatment. Holistic because it concentrates on the whole person and not on his illness or the symptoms of that illness—not even just on his feet. Hand in hand with this fundamental belief goes a working knowledge of anatomy and human biology, a certain insight into the patient's psycho-social environment and lifestyle, and an awareness of the significance and nature of his disease.

Powers of intuition, knowledge of people and therapeutic responsibility are not things that can be learned from a book. The greatest and best teacher is and will remain the practice itself.

Everyone who is interested in reflexology has the right to find out as much about it as he can. There is nothing magical or mysterious about it that makes it the property of a certain élite. All the basic essentials of reflexology, its premises and applications, are set out as clearly and concisely as possible in this book. We deal briefly with its history and principles, discuss the meaning of sickness and health, and give a detailed explanation of the zone system. In an appendix to the main text, which deals with reflex zone massage of the feet, there are illustrations showing the reflex zones of the hands. The chapter called 'Questions and Answers' gives quick answers to the most important questions raised by this method of treatment. The photographs at the back of the book supplement the graphic illustrations.

This book has arisen out of personal experience and conviction. We hope it will offer everyone who is interested the opportunity to find out about the principles of reflexology and perhaps benefit from putting into practice the methods described here.

We would like to stress once again that it is not our purpose to emphasize the differences between reflexology and orthodox medicine, but to find a common ground in shared knowledge. All our strivings towards a healthier world would be in vain if we aimed merely to replace one set of opinions with another. As the old Chinese proverb has it: 'The healer is right.'

It is in this spirit that we wish our readers much success and the patience necessary to achieve it.

Franz Wagner Ph.D.

Institute for Integrative Bodywork and
Psychological Counselling
A-4230 Pregarten
Austria

In the silence your heart knows the mystery of night and day.
But your ears thirst for the sound of knowledge.
You want to know in words what you have always known in your
soul . . .

The hidden spring must leap directly from your soul and flow
singing to the sea;
Then the treasure deep within you will become visible to your
eyes.
But do not weigh your unknown treasure on the scales;
And do not explore the depths of your knowledge with rod and
line
For the self is a bottomless infinite sea . . .

Khalil Gibran

1

Beginnings

The holistic approach of natural healing methods and reflex zone massage

The growing popularity of reflex zone massage is due to the fact that it is a method of helping oneself and others to an increased state of well-being, relaxation and inner harmony. It can be practised in almost any situation, it costs nothing and you need no equipment. There are only two provisos: the first is an exact knowledge of the reflex zones and the connections between them, and the second is a professional and spiritual integrity, a unity of thought and action crucial for anyone who works with people.

Only a few years ago the mere mention of healing methods like reflex zone massage was likely to cause an uproar among both doctors and patients. There was widespread uncertainty in both camps. Orthodox medicine kept its distance because reflexology could not be explained in terms of traditional methods or modes of thought. Patients were dubious because it was a type of treatment that demanded active participation from them and required them to rethink their attitude to their own bodies. But gradually, as reflexology proved itself to be successful, it won more and more converts. Doctors started to adopt its methods in their own practices, with beneficial results to their patients. Conferences on reflex zone therapy at medical training schools drew enthusiastic attendance. The fact that there is no successful explanation of how reflexology works does not dampen its success—indeed, the number of people prepared to admit that we still know far too little about mankind and that there are many things we are unable to understand or explain, is growing all the time.

If more and more people are turning to reflexology as a simple way of caring for their own health and well-being, it is because people are developing a new and responsible attitude to themselves, a new awareness of sickness and health that leads them increasingly to trust natural methods of healing and, at the same time, gives them more faith in themselves.

Doctors and therapists are now frequent attenders of weekend courses and conferences devoted to so-called alternative medicine. They want to be able to pass on what they learn to their patients, who are keen to discover natural health treatments that bring them into closer contact with the healer and have no dangerous side-effects. All the natural and holistic methods of healing are now gaining widespread public recognition, because it is at last being realized that they can and often do bring relief to those who are suffering, making long-term reliance on drugs a thing of the past.

From time to time natural therapy is ridiculed because it cannot be explained in conventional scientific terms, but if it helps its patients, then its methods are justified. We owe a great deal to scientific medical research, but in the end it is the individual, his feelings and his health that count, and medical science tends all too often to reduce the human patient to a laboratory statistic.

There are no miracle cures. When a cure succeeds beyond human expectation and imagination, it is because our assumptions about human biology are mistaken, or our knowledge of it is incomplete. 'Miracle cures' that seem beyond our comprehension merely serve to show how grossly we have underestimated the potential of the human organism.

We often underestimate the human body because we have forgotten how to read it, how to listen to it and interpret what it says to us. We have lost touch with our bodies. The body communicates in a way that is easy to understand, provided you know the language. Every one of us has to re-learn that language from the beginning. Our understanding of the body's language is progressing slowly, hand in hand with our understanding of the body as a whole.

As our understanding grows, it brings with it new concepts of sickness and health, new insight into what it means to be ill and to be well. Since the times of Hippocrates, health has been defined as a balanced state, and disease as imbalance. Healing a disease involves ousting an intruder so that order can be restored.

According to Paracelsus, nature is the greatest healer. Every medical cure can be traced to biological roots. The body's latent powers of healing are released and work to re-establish the equilibrium necessary for normal functioning. The power to heal lies in the body itself, though it may be buried or defused. We have lost the skill of mobilizing these healing forces—indeed, we are responsible for suppressing them. We have to learn all over again how to work with instead of against our bodies' natural powers of healing and defence, to support and nurture them instead of denying and stifling them.

Orthodox medicine aims primarily to eliminate the symptoms of disease. The holistic approach to healing says that we should work with and not against these manifestations of illness, as they are the natural expression of what is happening inside the body.

Admittedly conventional medicine can succeed in removing the manifestations of an illness—at least temporarily—much faster than other methods. But in so doing, conventional medicine also suppresses the body's natural powers of healing, often for so long that they cease to be able to function at all. We do not aim to question the effectiveness or the achievement of modern medicine in the West, but we do want to emphasize its one-sidedness. We are always glad when patients of orthodox medicine turn to reflexology for help, never more so than when their own doctors recommend it. In many such cases, and above all where patients are suffering from one or another kind of malfunction, reflex zone massage has taken over from and replaced formal medical treatment.

Holistic methods of healing—and reflex zone massage is one of them—do not isolate a disease and treat that alone, they treat the whole person. They do not work specifically on the impaired organ or the malfunctioning system, but always on the whole person. In this connection we must stress again that the intuitive skills of recognizing the roots of a patient's problem and working sympathetically with him are things that cannot be learned from this or any other book. The only way to learn is by experience, practice, self-knowledge and a constant attentiveness to the individual patient. It should not be assumed that knowledge alone can eliminate disease. Reflexology gives us the opportunity of understanding the body as a whole and learning how to help it mobilize its own powers of healing and defence to restore it to a healthy equilibrium.

Of course reflex zone massage is not a do-it-yourself way to instant health, as is sometimes implied in the popular press. It is a subject that needs to be approached seriously, something a well-known magazine was not prepared to do when it printed an article on reflexology under the title 'Tickle yourself to health—there's no funnier method of self-help'.

The principles of natural therapy

Healing the body should not involve forcing anything upon it that might contribute to its distress. The primary aim of the healer is to make the body receptive to healing. This is a principle that holds good across all ages and all cultural barriers. Every social community, every race had rituals that it enacted in the presence of anyone who was sick to create a climate in which healings could take place—a climate of solidarity, trust, openness, sharing, helping, not judging. Holistic methods of healing are totally open and start with the premise that we live in harmony with nature as we, along with all other forms of life, are creations of nature and can normally take care of ourselves in a natural way. In this sense, reflex zone massage can be said to be a natural method of healing, because it is derived from experience and constantly proves itself in practice.

There are four other basic principles for natural therapy:

1. The treatment must use natural means alone.
2. It must never cause the patient any harm.
3. It must be holistic.
4. It should stimulate the organism to release its own healing powers and work with them.

Only natural stimulants and remedies will provoke natural reactions in the body. These reactions will be long-lasting and have no harmful side-effects. Whereas orthodox medicine aims to trigger an immediate and quantifiable reaction, natural therapy works indirectly to activate the body's own healing powers and defences. The principles of holistic therapy state that it is impossible to treat disease in isolation. The manifestations of disease indicate that the organism has been disrupted and is working to cure itself and find a new balance. The seat of the disease may be in a different part of the body from the one in which it manifests itself. Illness should be understood in terms of the patient's whole life, as a crisis in his life, and not as a meaningless accident. Holistic therapists do not shirk this central human issue and their purpose is to help the patient to make the connection himself. This is the first step towards activating the patient's own healing powers and what is meant by working with the disease instead of trying to quash it. For us, the word 'therapy' does not mean so much a technique or method of treatment, as an attitude and approach to sickness and health.

The holistic approach to the life of the individual is that it is a process of continuing unfolding and developing and that sickness is an interruption of that process. This point of view was lost sight of for a long time in favour of a scientific, mechanical and thus one-sided approach to life. Only with the gradual breakdown of rigid traditional scientific theory could new ways be discovered of applying the ancient arts of healing to today's world and interpreting their message for modern society.

Medicine as a system of thought

The way in which we describe sickness, health, medicine or therapy, depends on our attitudes towards them. Language and thought are inextricably connected. The language we use and the words we choose not only reflect what we see, they also reveal what we overlook. For example, if Galileo had not thrown overboard Aristotle's theory of limited free fall in a swinging stone, he would never have come across the pendulum. What Galileo did was to perceive the same thing differently, and to use his own language to describe it. Then it made sense. Similarly, in medicine, if an inappropriate theory is used to explain a certain disorder, the probability is that the treatment prescribed will be equally inappropriate. In the final analysis, language marks the limits of our understanding, and we are hampered in our search for the truth unless we can throw off the chains of our linguistic limitations.

This explains why the success of reflex zone massage cannot be expressed in scientific terms. We are constantly made aware of this whenever we speak to doctors about the body's natural healing powers or the body's life forces. The introduction of new words into the vocabulary is clearly not a solution in itself—the words must be part of a whole system of thought. Medicine is not just medicine, irrespective of where and how it is applied; it is related to a cultural background, which has its own views, explanations and interpretations of mankind and the world.

At medical colleges and training centres there is often a sense that we know all there is to know about medicine. This is a great stumbling block, as knowledge alone cannot cure the patient. Experience and understanding should be brought to bear along with intuition and sympathy for each individual as a whole person.

Broadly speaking there are two distinct systems of thought in medicine today:

1. Western medicine aims to diagnose diseases and eradicate

them by implementing changes in the body. Two of its main areas of concern are the organs and the blood. It is based on anatomy (a study of the structure of the body) and histology (a study of the body tissue). It is above all a physically orientated science (somatic medicine).

2. Alternative medicines have their roots mostly in Far Eastern cultures and are concerned primarily with processes, dynamics and energy. This means that they deal with malfunctions and disorders that are very often outside the province of Western scientific medicine. It is important that the two systems are not seen as competing against each other, but as complementary.

Our health is influenced by many factors. They may be important or seemingly trivial; they may be physical, emotional or psychological. Today, more than ever before, our health is also affected by the environment in which we live. All these factors should be seen in connection with one another, as each one influences the next. The awareness of these inter-connecting factors enables holistic therapists to look further than the symptoms of a disease, down into its deeper structure.

This process of penetration is reminiscent of the healing methods of the Far East, but it must be more than just the borrowing of a technique, or it will end up being merely a pale imitation of Far Eastern practices. Far more than this, it is a different way of thinking, of talking about oneself and of seeing oneself and the world. In this sense reflex zone massage is a holistic form of therapy, which is always concerned to see the patient as a whole, to understand him and treat his whole being.

Sickness and health

Today there is a general lack of understanding about the true nature of illness and the healing process, because the mechanical, physical and chemical explanations available tell us nothing about the human factor. The most important consideration in the understanding of disease is not the biophysical and chemical reactions in the body, but the human nature of the human being. An almost exclusively scientific approach has reduced the patient to a set of statistics. These methods are of course excellent for technical purposes, but are hardly suited to furthering our knowledge about human beings. Many of the holistic therapies renounce scientific criteria altogether, on the grounds that they are narrow and often contradictory. Humanity transcends the narrow boundaries laid down by scientific thought. Healing processes are not necessarily scientific—though they may be, or become so. This does not detract from their ability to heal—on the contrary, it says far more about which aspects of human nature can be scientifically understood, and which cannot.

For the purposes of orthodox scientific medicine the human body is an object. Knowledge about it is scientifically exact, but scientific methods alone cannot comprehend humanity, any more than they can measure man's soul or his emotions. Having said this, we should not make the mistake of rejecting scientific medicine in favour of non-scientific medicine; we must rather consider all the available forms of therapy with a new understanding and a new awareness.

Truly therapeutic thinking and treatment springs from a knowledge of human nature and not, in the first instance, from a knowledge of disease. Scientific development and an increasingly detailed knowledge of the body's smallest components, the cells, whose workings can now be explained and understood, has thrust the body and its physical functions into the foreground and completely discounted the spirit and the emotions. Man's wholeness and oneness disappeared in a minute scrutiny of his parts. What we must do now is to restore the balance and perspective to our view of man.

Illnesses are traditionally regarded as deviations from the normal state of things, as disruption to the process of life. They are defined as essentially negative phenomena that limit or break down the body's functions. We should like to consider the nature of disease as a process happening to the patient. This will help the therapist in his treatment of the disease, or, to put it more accurately in his treatment of the patient.

In dealing with the concepts of sickness and health, we have to reach beyond technical schemes of thought about the human body to living thought about man himself. The human organism is in a state of constant change and renewal. Sickness and health are not fixed or permanent commodities; similarly there are no fixed starting points or finishing points for therapy—its beginning and end cannot be pre-determined. Life itself is change, growth, movement. This is why we must address ourselves first of all to those life forces that promote continued health in the body and attempt to stimulate them, by massaging reflex zones on the feet, to releasing a flow of creative energy that will restore the body to harmony.

Forces at work in the cosmos are also at work in man—he too is a theatre for cosmic energy. When the play of energy is harmonic, man is said to be well; when the field of energy becomes a theatre of war, he is ill. These forces are given different names in different languages, cultures and systems of thought, but whether they are called yin and yang or sympathetic and parasympathetic is ultimately immaterial. The principle remains the same—we are talking about equilibrium and harmony, a balance created by tension and relaxation.

Thus we must seek a new understanding of health, as well as a new way of looking at disease. The spread of confidence in natural methods of healing has coincided with a revolution in our attitude towards health. Whereas traditional medicine is primarily concerned with overcoming symptoms and healing disease, alternative medicine and methods of self-help aim above all to maintain health. Alternative therapy sets out to care actively for the patient's health and preserve order; what it does not do is to wait passively for harmony to fall into disorder, a term also used by the orthodox medical profession. In view of this, we must never lose sight of the fact that there is no such thing as 'disease', there is only the sick person. We are concerned with the fate, the life of the individual and his vital energies, which can be balanced, or more or less disordered. This is the subject of our treatment, and not 'a cold', or 'a headache'.

In spite of its huge potential and the wide-ranging success it has enjoyed so far, reflex zone massage of the feet should not be regarded as a universal panacea. Neither is it primarily a method of diagnosis. Although we do deal with disorder and its roots in a holistic sense, the greatest achievement of reflexology lies in the mobilization and harmonization of the body's natural powers of healing.

From our own experience we can safely say that the prejudices of traditional medicine towards our actually very simple methods of treatment are fast disappearing. Therapists and people who work in the health services who attend our courses report increasingly successful collaboration with doctors who have seen with their own eyes that reflexology works and want to find out more about it. Medical conferences often hear from doctors who have themselves applied reflex zone therapy to their patients' feet, often with a radical improvement in their own relationship to the patient as well as in the patient's condition.

It should be said again that criticism of the inadequacies of clinical medicine is not the purpose of this book, nor is it our wish to advocate its replacement by reflexology. Criticism and dissatisfaction with medicine are as old as medicine itself. However, criticism in recent times has struck a new note, which says that medicine, like modern society itself, has developed far enough. It seems to have come to a natural halt and what we hear now is Nature, clamouring to be listened to once more. Technological advance has put our natural environment at risk, and it is also endangering human nature. Man as a whole living being has become more and more fragmented in the wake of scientific progress. The obstacles to understanding that face us now cannot be overcome unless we change our point of view, expand our consciousness and enlarge our horizons.

Most of the well-known branches of so-called alternative medicine achieve this by looking back, often thousands of years, to a treasured legacy of thought. Common to all of them is a certain understanding of the world, of human nature and of disease. They have a shared view of humanity—such a view is lacking in modern medicine, just as it has no concept of health, only a rather limited theory of disease. At the 1982 Conference on Humanism in Salzburg, specialists from various disciplines gathered together to discuss the question 'How sick is modern medicine?' and proposed a motion that declared: 'We don't need a new medical system—what we need is a new view of mankind!'

Working with reflex zone therapy of the feet, we must always bear in mind that we are working with a whole person, and not restrict our attention to one aspect of him, his symptoms, or his illness. Naturally we cannot always take absolutely everything into account (the influence of his surroundings, the conditions at his place of work and so on), but we can do much to avoid adding to his problems if we treat him as a human being.

The apparent simplicity of applying reflex zone therapy to the feet and hands should not be underestimated. Reflex zone massage should not be seen merely as a technique that can be applied mechanically according to the principles of classical massage. Reflexology is not a different technique; it is more than that—it is a different form of treatment. It is not sufficient to probe the soles of the feet at random and hope for the best. After all, you would not expect to make an aircraft fly simply pulling a few levers. This is no different.

Anyone can copy a technique, but its effects will depend on the attitude of the person performing the action. How a technique is applied also depends on the cultural background and origins of the therapy, on the relationship between the therapist and the patient, and on the attitude of both to life to general. Finally, the success of reflex zone therapy, as of any other method of healing, including orthodox medicine, depends on the professional and personal integrity and responsibility of the therapist.

2

History and Track Record

About the history of reflex zone therapy

The practice of massaging the reflex zones of the feet comes from ancient folk medicine. It is known to have been employed by Red Indian tribes and was probably passed down to us by the Incas, who greatly refined the old Indian techniques. Writers of ancient Rome also describe healing methods that correspond exactly to our concept of reflex zones. Bascially, then, our knowledge about the reflex zones of the feet and how to massage them for the purposes of therapy has been handed down to us over the course of thousands of years.

Awareness of the body's reflexes and how to use them is found in many cultures. The ancient Chinese developed the technique of acupressure, the roots of which lie in the knowledge of reflex zones and the relationships between them. Indian and Indonesian healers also made reference to the reflex zones in the feet and hands.

Fighting pain has always been a major human preoccupation. In India and China, the treatment of pain at certain pressure points of the body was practised over 5,000 years ago. Today the most highly developed and perhaps strongest branch of this ancient form of therapy is acupuncture ('acus' is Latin for 'needle'). In Central Europe very similar methods were described by Drs Adamus and A'Tatis in 1580, and in Leipzig at about the same time Dr Ball published a book about his methods of indirect treatment—by exerting pressure at certain points he was able to cure disease and relieve pain in other parts of the body. History tells, too, how the famous Florentine sculptor, Benvenuto Cellini (1500–1571), suffered a great deal of pain and was treated for it by vigorous massage of both hands and feet. The twentieth President of the United States, President Garfield (1831–1881), suffered extreme pain after an assassination attempt and when all other remedies had failed he tried foot massage, which turned out to be the only method of treatment that brought him any relief.

Today, reflex zone massage is still practised in its original form by Indians living on reserves in America. They use it to heal disease, but primarily as a method of relieving pain.

Though it cannot be proved, specialists tend to agree that it was Dr William Fitzgerald who first came across zone therapy as practised by the Red Indians, and it is to his observations and studies that we owe our modern concepts of reflexology.

Zone therapy according to Dr Fitzgerald

Dr William Henry Fitzgerald (1872–1942) was an American doctor who developed the zone theory named after him and published his findings on this form of healing in 1913.

Dr Fitzgerald studied at the University of Vermont, from which he graduated in 1895. He then practised medicine for two and a half years in Boston City Hospital, before moving to the Central London Ear, Nose and Throat Hospital. He also spent two years in Vienna at the ear, nose and throat clinic there under the famous Professors Politzer and Chiari.

He made his findings about zone therapy available to medical science while he was head of the ear, nose and throat department of St Francis Hospital, Connecticut. He had discovered that pressure and massage, when applied to certain zones or points on the body, could improve the function of the internal organs and relieve pain, sometimes causing it to disappear completely. The distance between the organ where the effect of the treatment took place, and the area that was treated was immaterial.

One story about Dr Fitzgerald claims that he hit upon the idea of zone therapy after performing certain experiments on his patients. The story goes that he made minute surgical incisions in their flesh and observed that they reacted very differently to the anticipated pain. Those with a low threshold of pain gripped the arms of the chair they were sitting in and dug their fingers into its upholstery. Dr Fitzgerald took this observation and investigated the concept behind it—that pressure points on the body have reflective connections in other areas. This, it is said, is how he rediscovered the methods of therapy used thousands of years ago by the ancient Chinese and called acupressure.

Whether it happened in this way or not, Dr Fitzgerald developed a new zone system particular to his own concept of the ancient therapy. His observations and discoveries about the human body led him to divide it into ten zones, which run from the top of the head to the tips of the toes. This zone system has

The zones of the body according to Dr Fitzgerald

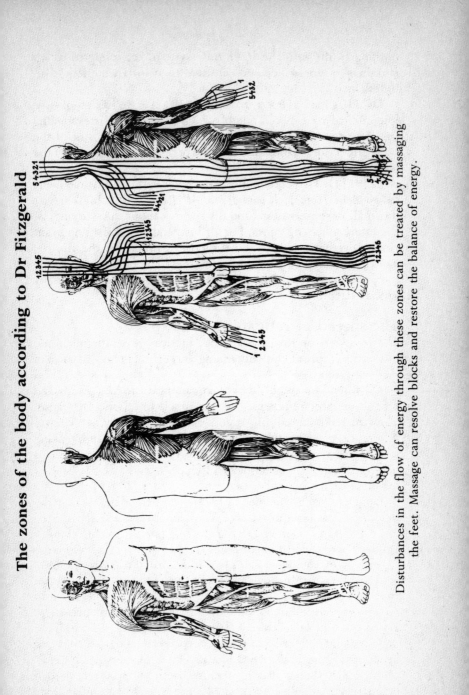

Disturbances in the flow of energy through these zones can be treated by massaging the feet. Massage can resolve blocks and restore the balance of energy.

nothing to do with the head zone system, according to which certain skin zones become sensitive to pain when there is an illness involving the internal organs.

Dr Fitzgerald's body zones consist of two series of five longitudinal zones, each one of which ends in the corresponding finger or toe. Everything that happens in a specific zone of the body affects and is influenced by the organs and other parts of the body within that zone.

In 1917 Dr Fitzgerald published a book with Dr Edwin Bowers called *Zone Therapy, Relieving Pain At Home*. In this book he set down all his observations and discoveries about the workings of the interconnecting zones. For Dr Fitzgerald the most important zones for therapeutic stimulation were found on the fingers, hands, lips, tongue, gums, nose and toes. The reflex zones of the feet, so crucial for modern therapy, were not singled out for any special attention.

The spread of reflexology
The followers of zone therapy in America grew in number and interest in it spread, not only among the general public, but also in medical circles.

J.S. Riley MD and his wife were amongst the most renowned practitioners of reflexology, doing much to advance its cause. They treated hundreds of patients with zone therapy, working on different zones of the body with great success and making valuable new discoveries at the same time. Dr Riley is perhaps best known as the teacher of Mrs Eunice Ingham, who assisted in his practice for a number of years.

Eunice Ingham, who died in 1974, documented her work in the field of reflexology in two well-known books, *Stories the Feet can Tell* (1938) and *Stories the Feet have Told* (1963). In this context another book worth mentioning is *Helping Yourself with Foot Reflexology* by the American physiotherapist, M. Carter (1969).

According to Mrs Ingham, reflex zone therapy is a massage treating pressure points on the feet with a special grip technique—an action of the thumb that could 'reduce sugar crystals to a powder'. Mrs Ingham posed a theory of 'crystalline deposits' and believed that the success of reflexology lay above all in 'freezing the body from blockages in the nervous system'. Today this theory has generally been supplanted, though practitioners often use these simple terms to explain reflexology to their patients.

We know today that the workings of reflexology are altogether more subtle, deep and complicated than was suspected before and that no direct cause-and-effect-type explanation or linear model can sufficiently explain them. Our own ongoing investigations into the subject, particularly in conjunction with a university hospital and using EEG machines to chart patients' physiological reactions, has made it clear that there is no simple answer to the question: How does reflexology work?

There are many explanations for its success and these vary according to the research and experience of the therapist and his knowledge of other branches of science. We cannot come to a final conclusion about how the therapy works, but we are happy with our extremely positive findings and our experience of it. Two things that are beyond doubt, however, are that it does work and that we know how best to apply it for optimum results. The direct connections between the various reflex zones are obvious as a result of the success of reflexology, even though to date no anatomical connections between the zones massaged and areas affected have been proved. It seems that we are dealing with phenomena that simply cannot be explained on the physical plane. We regard the workings of reflexology as a holistic expression of the forces of life.

In some cases, the theory of 'crystalline deposits' can help to explain what happens. When the metabolism is not functioning properly, uric acid and excess calcium are among the waste products that build up in the body. Large deposits of these substances cannot be dispersed by the normal activity of the endocrine system. By massaging the reflex zones on the feet we aim to reverse this damming-up process so that the deposits become absorbed into the blood and lymph and are eventually eliminated from the body.

For most practical purposes the concept that best explains how reflexology works is this: that stimulating the feet through massage works like acupressure to activate a flow of energy that courses through the body in meridinal zones.

Another way of looking at it is that each one of the 72,000 nerve endings in the foot is connected with other parts of the body and that massaging these nerve endings sends impulses to those areas.

For the purposes of reflexology, we could think of the body as a hologram; within this hologram each of the millions of cells would be a further hologram. Each cell would carry the basic information about all the other cells and about the whole body.

Recent developments

The British healer Robert St John has developed a prenatal therapy based on the principles of reflexology and his own experience of working with patients. His belief that illness is created by the patient has led him to concentrate on the very first formative phase of life in the womb. He believes that all disability is caused by blocking, and that it manifests itself in two very different ways. On the one hand, the subject may be severely cut off from life, and on the other, thrust too violently into it. Autistic and mongoloid children are clear extremes of these two aspects of blocking.

As none of the usual methods of treatment took his theory into account, St John began working more intensively with reflexology, and he realized that most physical disabilities correspond to a blockage in the reflex zone of the spine. He also found that his treatment had the same effect when he confined it to the reflex zones of the spine and did not treat the other zones on the feet.

He then turned his attention to the psychological aspects of the treatment. In the heel he located the reflex zone of the spine that corresponds to the maternal principle, and in the first joint of the big toe he located the paternal principle. He came to the conclusion that the line connecting these two points would reflect the gestation period, and the reflex zones of the spine could therefore be seen as reflex zones in time.

He does not regard life in the womb as a part of the past that is lost to us, but as an integral part of our present experience. Everything that is happening to us in the present is the coming to fruition of an energy pattern that was established while we were still in the womb.

Prenatal therapy—or metamorphic practice, as it is also known—is now practised all over the world. Further progress in this area has been made by Robert St John's most famous pupil, Gaston St Pierre. While reflexology aims primarily to treat physical disturbances, the future of prenatal therapy is in exploring the psychological configuration behind the time-map of our life in the womb, as revealed by the spinal zones on the feet. The metamorphosis practitioner concentrates on the potential latent in this time span—the potential of the individual's whole life. In the same way that the earth nurtures the seed, encouraging it to put down a root and develop into a plant, metamorphosis provides the wherewithal in the realm of time for life, growth, development and the fulfilment of individual potential.

The ultimate goal of everyone is self-realization—the acorn grows into an oak tree, the caterpillar is transformed into a butterfly and each human individual becomes himself. Metamorphosis works beyond time and space in the realm of energy potential: it deals with the transformation of what we are into what we can be. The success of this form of therapy goes to show that the scope of treatment is as unlimited as the potential of life itself.

These developments in reflexology seem to have the same inner logic noticeable in other natural forms of treatment, such as homoeopathy. There, too, it is impossible to apply strictly rational empirical criteria because what the healer is dealing with is fields of energy and the patterns they create. In fact, if we are honest, it must be admitted that there can be no ultimate explanation for the workings of the human organism and that the possibilities for interpretation are as many and various as human beings themselves. The whole universe is made of energy, life is energy, and what we are dealing with in this context is energy too, whether we are able to understand the laws of that energy or not. Life is the greatest healer of all.

If you would like to know more about metamorphosis, write to The Metamorphic Association, 67 Ritherdon Road, London SW17 8QE.

3
The Zone System

How the body is divided up into zones
What we see on the feet is a mirror image of the human being itself, body and soul. We can use the feet like a map. In reflexology the feet are the most reliable guide, though we should not make the mistake of concentrating on them alone.

According to Dr Fitzgerald's zone therapy, the body is divided into ten longitudinal zones. The zones on this grid extend into the feet, which are also divided into ten zones. The grid lines run from the scalp to the soles of the feet, and down the arms to the fingers, Exactly how these zones were delineated in the first place is uncertain, but the system remains a great help in orientating zones on the feet for massage.

The longitudinal divisions are crossed by a further set of lateral divisions. This allows us to plot a two-dimensional map of the body on the feet. If you take the time to become acquainted with

Lateral zone	Location	Organs	Referral area on the foot
A	shoulder girdle	organs of the head and neck	toes
B	diaphragm	organs of the chest and upper abdomen	metatarsals, Lisfranc's joint line
C	pelvic floor	organs of the abdomen and pelvis	tarsus, ankle joint

the anatomy of the feet, to feel them for yourself in every little detail, you will be amazed how little you knew of these intricate masterpieces of construction.

From the diagrams on pages 38 and 39 you will see that the horizontal zones are easy to locate and correspond to natural anatomical divisions. The body is divided vertically and horizontally into zones, and each one has its corresponding reflective zone on the feet. By using the zones on the feet, we can treat the organs in those zones on the body.

Two examples:

1. **The spine** (*columna vertebralis*) is found on the body grid running down either side of zone 1. In the feet, it runs all along the inside edge of both feet through the horizontal zones A, B and C.
2. **The lungs** (*pulmones*) are a paired organ located in body zones 1–5 in the second horizontal zone. From this we find the reflex zone of the lungs in the area of the fifth metatarsal above Lisfranc's joint line (longitudinal zones 1–5 and lateral zone B).

The significance of the zones

Reflexology is not intended to implement a mechanical cure from without, but to activate and harmonize the body's own life forces and healing powers. In massaging the reflex zones of the feet we are massaging tissue, and we are working along the meridians of acupuncture. But these facts are incidental to our purpose, which is to stimulate a particular zone on the foot to send an impulse to a corresponding part of the body, where it will take effect. The reflective connections between various parts of the body are well known to orthodox medicine. Head's zone system, for example, describes areas of skin that are connected to certain internal organs. If these organs become diseased, the corresponding areas of skin show extreme sensitivity to pain.

Reflexology is based on the zone theory and understands the term 'reflex' to mean the 'reflection' of the organs and different parts of the body projected in miniature on the feet. Such projections are not only to be found on the soles of the feet, but also on the tops and along the inside and outside as far up as just above the ankle. There are also reflex zones on the hands, nose and ears.

It cannot be overstressed that we are concerned with zones, and not with fixed points. The exact location and extent of the zones differs according to the constitution of each individual. The

Anatomy of the foot—dorsal view

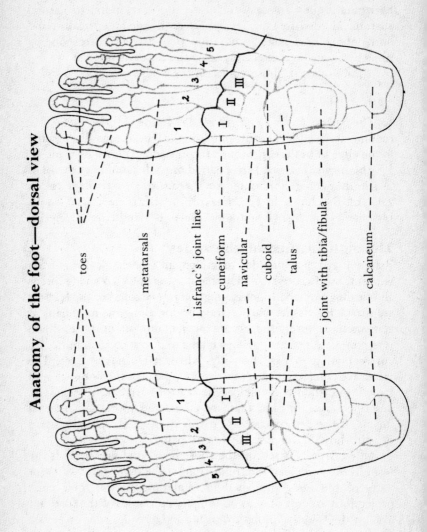

toes

metatarsals

Lisfranc's joint line

cuneiform

navicular

cuboid

talus

joint with tibia/fibula

calcaneum

Anatomy of the foot—the sole

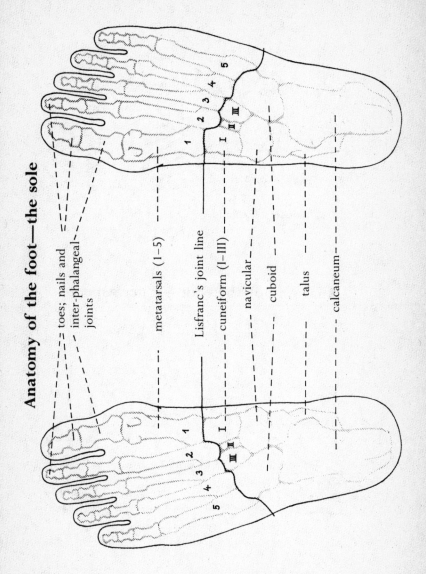

toes; nails and
inter-phalangeal
joints

metatarsals (1–5)

Lisfranc's joint line

cuneiform (I–III)

navicular

cuboid

talus

calcaneum

Anatomy of the foot—outer aspect

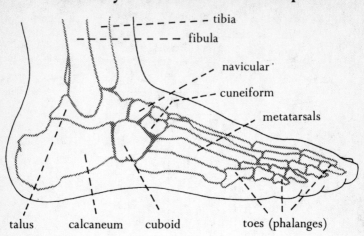

talus calcaneum cuboid toes (phalanges)

tibia
fibula
navicular
cuneiform
metatarsals

Anatomy of the foot—inner aspect

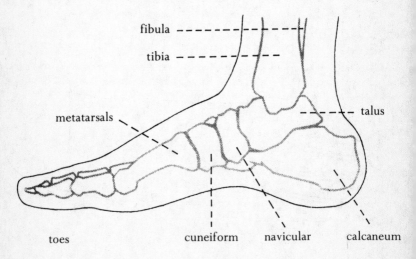

fibula
tibia
talus
metatarsals
toes cuneiform navicular calcaneum

The foot—the body's support

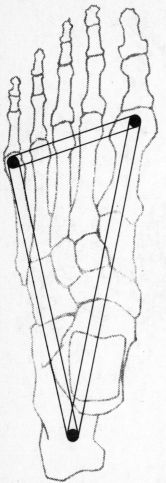

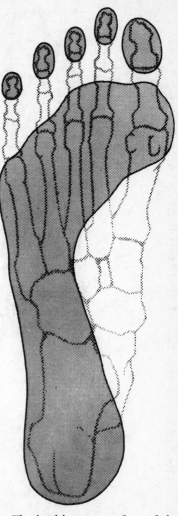

The structure of
the foot, showing how the
body's weight presses upon it

The load-bearing surface of the
foot is cushioned for protection

The feet as a mirror of the two halves of the body

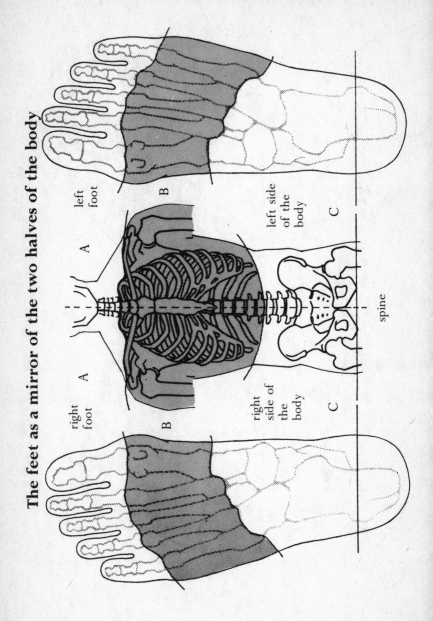

right
foot

A

A

left
foot

B

B

right
side of
the
body

C

left side
of the
body

C

spine

Corresponding longitudinal and lateral zones in the body and the foot

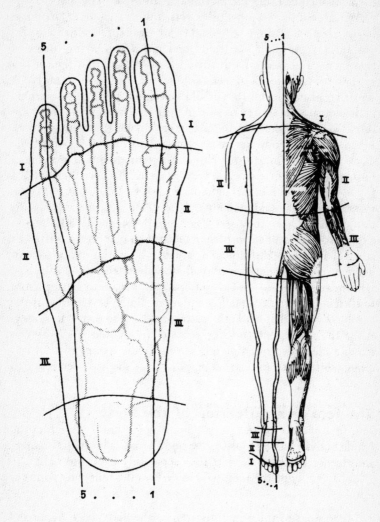

right foot—sole   body—back view

zones are not strictly defined, and their boundaries cannot be universally applied. They are areas that interleave or overlap, and it must be left to the experienced hand of the therapist to discover them manually, using his tactile and intuitive experience.

We should like to repeat that reflexology encounters pain in a positive spirit. Pain is the nightwatchman of health, a guard standing at the door—a friend and not a foe. Many forms of treatment are based on a distorted view of pain: they fight it as a symptom of illness. In reflexology we see it differently. A sensitive place on the foot is like an alarm going off—warning bells indicate the source of pain in the body. It would be absurd to think we could shut off the alarm and make the pain go away.

An example from our own practice illustrates this point. One day a woman came to our clinic. She had already undergone a number of examinations and tests to try to discover the root of a vague illness she felt throughout her body. As she got on to the massage table she said jokingly that her teeth were the only healthy things about her, they gave her no problems at all. But an exploratory examination of her feet told a completely different story. The only real problem seemed to be in the reflex zone of her teeth. Treatment was immediately directed at this zone and within a matter of hours the patient began to suffer from toothache and took herself to a dental clinic. The source of the trouble was hidden while the pain spread to the rest of her body. After this treatment and her visit to the dentist, the patient's trouble cleared up completely, even to the extent that she no longer suffered from the rheumatic attacks she had been prone to before.

The feet as a reflection of the body

The feet should be seen as a pair, a single unity reflecting the whole body. Thus we look for the body's map in both feet at once, and do not think of the left foot separately from the right.

When studying the feet, we should bear the following points in mind:

1. According to the zonal division of the body, each organ and part of the body can be located on the foot in the corresponding zone. The size of the zone often depends on the size of the corresponding organ.
2. The reflex zones on the feet are sited according to the anatomy of the body—for example, the heart is behind the lobe of the lungs.

3. The right half of the body is reflected in the right foot, and the left half in the left foot.

4. Paired organs, such as the lungs, kidneys and ovaries, are to be found one in each foot. Single organs, such as the heart and liver are to be found in either the left or the right foot according to their anatomical position.

5. The position of the organs and the parts of the body is also reflected in the zones of the feet. Central organs, such as the oesophagus, are found on the insides of the feet, and outer parts of the body, such as the shoulder joint, are found on the outside.

6. Reflex zones of the organs, which are central to the material in this book, are more easily accessible from the soles of the feet. Nerves, muscles and bones are more easily treated from the top or back (dorsal side) of the feet.

4

The Principles of Reflex Zone Massage

The attitude of the therapist

Sometimes the desire to help a patient can be too strong, and the will to improve or cure his or her condition becomes a driving force that takes over the whole of the therapy. Physical and emotional tension on the part of the therapist carry over into his work and are in themselves blocks that can obstruct the natural effects of the message.

In the *Bhagavadgita* we read: 'Let the work in hand be your sole occupation—do not consider its fruits.' This is certainly true for reflexology. We are not pursuing the goal of eradicating disease or its symptoms. At the centre of our therapy is the patient himself, and we rely wholly on his life forces for our effectiveness. We should be able to communicate this trust to the patient.

Many people are only too ready to seek help from outside and never think of taking responsibility for themselves. The most positive attitude for the therapist is one of unlimited, undoubting trust in the powers of healing and powers of self-help of his patient, and this should not be clouded by a will to succeed. This attitude can do much for the self-determination of the person seeking help. When someone is in the position of seeking help, he is very vulnerable and very easily influenced. It is the simplest thing in the world to make the mistake of putting our own viewpoint to him and persuading him that we are right.

No matter how great his experience or knowledge of people, the therapist's point of view has its limitations and in the ultimate analysis only the patient can say what is right. We must concentrate on dissolving the blocks and allowing the energy to flow, otherwise the determination of the therapist could clash with the life forces of his patient, resulting in a stalemate.

If the therapist does find that no progress is made, he should ask himself whether his own attitude to his work is the right one. Reflexology, after all, does not work according to a set of preconceived ideas, nor do we take on ourselves personal responsibility for the patient's development or cure—what we are doing is to create the opportunity for the patient's own powers of healing to become effective, by releasing them and supporting their action.

The position of the patient

The correct positioning of the patient is an important factor in the success of reflexology. The most important points to observe apply to other kinds of massage as well:

1. Provide a soft and comfortable couch for the patient to lie on, perferably with adjustable head and foot rests.
2. Put cushions under the neck and knees to support a relaxed position.
3. The treatment should be carried out in a light, quiet, friendly room that is warm and well-ventilated, or somewhere where the patient feels at home, such as his own house.
4. Give the patient sufficient time to lie in a comfortable, relaxed position. Give yourself enough room to work without feeling cramped.

The patient should make himself as comfortable as possible (no tight clothing; a blanket if he likes). Clothes that restrict the breathing, such as bras and corsets, should be taken off. If patients have difficulty relaxing the feet before a massage, provide a blanket. With the blanket over them they will find that their feet naturally turn outwards in a relaxed position.

The best position for massage is lying down. If the patient is sitting, the angles of the hip and knee joints will prove a great hindrance. The patient's legs should be higher than his bottom, and his back should be raised so that eye-contact with the therapist, which is so vital for a trusting relationship, can be maintained. This is also important so that the therapist can read the patient's reactions, which will direct him in the form of his treatment.

The massage grip

The only tool needed for reflexology is a pair of hands. 'Tool' suggests something rather technical. But the massage grip has by its very nature nothing to do with the technical or the mechanical, nor with the pressure suggested by those terms. The use of the hands here, as elsewhere in human behaviour, is an expression of giving and taking, a symbol for personal relationship.

The movements of the hands in massage are dynamic and flowing; furthermore, they are infinitely suited in scope to the treatment of the feet. In contact between the hands and the feet, the feet should remain relaxed, and the hands should accommodate themselves to the feet. The feet are not rigid fixed objects—together with the hands they form a single unity in the work of reflexology.

Although the whole hand is enormously important in massage, the thumb needs particular consideration. The end of the thumb is the point of contact through which the dynamic energy of the hand flows to stimulate the healing reflexes. This is one of the main differences between reflex zone massage and ordinary mechanical massage.

The therapist presses the end of his thumb into the tissue of the patient's foot with a force suited to the individual patient, in a movement both relaxed and dynamic. The thumb should be neither bent nor completely straight, but supple and flowing in its movements, like the progress of a caterpillar. Not for nothing is this particular movement known as thumb-walking. It is characterized by a continuing alternation between tension and relaxation, or what can be called an active phase, penetrating and probing into the tissue of the foot, and a passive phase, in which the thumb draws back to its starting position. As the thumb withdraws, the massaging hand moves automatically and rhythmically forwards. This dynamic rhythmic massage harmonizes the flow of energy in the tissue it is treating.

The hand always moves forwards as the massage progresses and it aids the flowing movement of skin contact between hand and foot if never interrupted. The thumb is never bent to its full extent, because this hard angular movement would be a strain for the therapist and cause a tensing in the patient—not to mention having the therapist's thumb-nail digging into his foot.

As soon as you put it into practice, you will realize that the massage grip that works best is one which is accommodating and pliable. It should be able to adapt to different circumstances and meet different requirements as they arise, varying the therapeutic stimulation according to the disorder and the sensitivity of the patient.

For the masseur of the reflex zones, the hand is not merely a tool, it is a sensitive receptor of feeling and a means of communication between therapist and patient. The sensitive powers of the hand are an important aspect of the work of every

Recommended direction of massage strokes

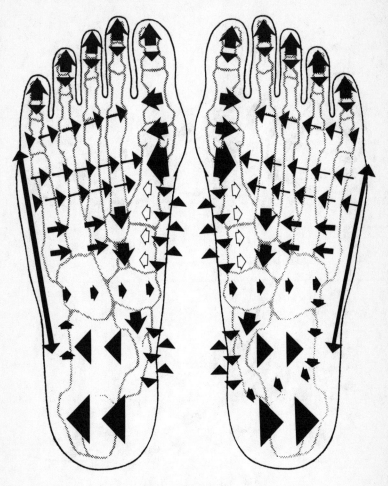

The soles of the feet

Recommended direction of massage strokes

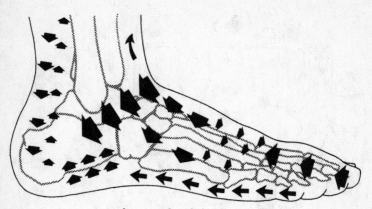

the outside of the foot

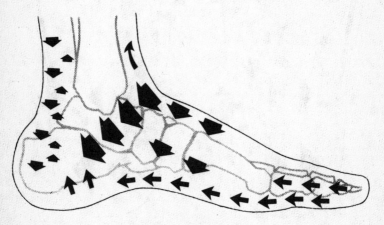

the inside of the foot

therapist, and one that is refined and developed as the therapist becomes more experienced.

There is no general standard by which to measure the tempo of the massage or the intensity of pressure—only practice can teach these things, and you eventually come to know them, literally, in your bones.

At the beginning of a reflex zone massage the masseur should proceed with special care and direct his attention particularly to the patient's reactions, which will be valuable in directing him how to continue.

The normal 'dynamic' massage has two main functions:

1. Activating (toning, strengthening).
A strong rhythmic, wave-like massage harmonizes the energies flowing through the referral zone and improves its functioning.
2. Passifying (calming, soothing).
A strong, constant and unmoving thumb pressure for 1–2 minutes has a calming and relaxing effect, especially with acute disturbances to the body's system such as colic, neuralgia, haemorrhaging and toothache, and with nervous disorders and over-tense muscles.

The order in which the zones are worked during a massage is not important. The direction of the massage will develop naturally and the order of treatment is usually determined by proximity of zones rather than anything else.

Beginning treatment

With the patient reclining comfortably as previously described, the therapist should sit, preferably on a swivel stool, upright and relaxed within easy reach of the patient's feet. He should never take the patient's feet onto his lap. The patient's position should make it possible for him to just let the massage happen, and to open himself up to the treatment from within—he should not be given the impression that he is helpless in the hands in the therapist. The patient should always feel that he can withdraw, which in this case means that he can withdraw his feet.

The first physical contact (after eye-contact and conversation) occurs when the therapist moves his hands over the patient's feet in a stroking motion. Stroking the patient's feet helps to build trust between patient and therapist, and it also gives the therapist the following important information about the feet:

1. Temperature.
2. Static build-up.
3. Muscle tone and tissue tone.
4. Skin condition.

In the first session of treatment the therapist tries to get as comprehensive a view of his patient as he can. The first session is investigative and exploratory. The means of investigation are sight and touch. The visual investigation is secondary. It does not act independently, but as a back-up for the physical investigation.

As the therapist works systematically through the reflex zones on the feet, he alternates the exploratory probing with further stroking movements to relax the patient and strengthen his thrust. The therapist notes down important discoveries for his files, so that he can easily refresh his memory about the patient before subsequent visits. Any records that he makes should never prevent the responsible practitioner from asking the patient each time how he feels, so that he always has fresh first-hand information. The patient's attitude and his reactions will be changing constantly, and written case notes serve only as a prompt.

Each individual's feet are quite different, revealing characteristics peculiar to that person. The personal aspect is one of the most fascinating things about reflexology. As you learn more, through course work or from your own experience, about how to read and interpret the personal language of the feet, you will realize that feet are never boring, and that in them is the whole life history of the person, waiting to be discovered.

The best way to understand a patient is to find out how he feels and, if you listen closely enough, he will tell you himself. He will give you the key to his healing. Ken Dychtwald has written in his book *Körperbewusstsein* (*Body Consciousness*) that our personal being and attitude to life is dependent not only on how well our bodies are functioning, but also on the way in which they are formed and structured. In Alexander Lowen's book *Bioenergetik* (*Bioenergetics*), we read that man is the sum of his experience; every single experience he has is stored in his personality and his body. Just as a tree feller can read the story of a tree from its annual rings, so it is possible to read the story of a man's life from his body.

After a certain amount of practice the student of reflexology will be able to see his success and the progress he has made, and it is a wonderful feeling to know that success is, quite literally, in your own hands.

Now we turn to the visual examination of the patient's feet, which will give information about:

1. Bone structure.
2. Skin condition.
3. The condition of the tissue.

The bone structure of the foot is remarkable in that it bears the weight of the whole body. From osteopathy and orthopaedics we know the importance of dynamic equilibrium in the bone structure of the foot. Abnormalities and deformities can cause blockages that give rise to considerable disturbance in the reflex zones of the feet. For example, a flattened transverse arch can affect the reflex zone to the shoulder girdle and the respiratory organs.

Every anatomical abnormality of the bones in the feet must result in a disturbance in the reflex zones around it. If the deformity is obvious, such as hallux valgus (see the colour plate section), then even a visual examination will be able to detect potential problems in the neck and the cervical spine in particular. A visual examination of the condition of the tissue can often given a clear indication of lymphatic blockages (for example, poor tissue condition in the area of the ankle or the basal joints of the toes indicates problems with the pelvis and chest respectively).

The condition of the skin is one of the most important sources of visual information. Changes of skin condition are not as important for the purposes of reflexology as the places at which those changes occur. The position of warts, athlete's foot, blisters, corns, cracked skin, flaking skin, varicose veins, callouses and scars, as well as the shape of each individual toe-nail, can tell the therapist much about the disorders of the patient's body.

Varicose veins and areas infected with verrucas should not be massaged. Varicose veins may be further damaged and the massage of verrucas will encourage them to spread to other parts of the feet and may also infect the therapist. Verrucas should be treated by a chiropodist.

It is important that the patient does not visit a chiropodist before his first reflexology session, or many important clues as to his condition may be eliminated.

The 'language' of the feet
The feet are not only a mirror of our current condition and of our development, they are also a symbol of our mobility and of the

connection of our life's progress with the movements of the universe. In Tao-te-king we read, 'There, where your feet stand, begins the journey of a thousand miles.' The feet carry the image of our selves and our relationship with the world. They can tell how we are and how we regard ourselves. We talk of 'weak footings' and 'strong footings', of 'standing on your own two feet' and 'having both feet on the ground'. All these ways of talking about the feet symbolize a certain attitude to oneself and the world. We are connected by our feet to the ground; our feet are also a connection between our earthly and spiritual life. The feet play a special part in many religions—we have only to think of the washing of Jesus' feet. Through our feet we remain in constant contact with the outside world.

Thousands of years ago the Chinese developed the idea that different parts of the body represent different contacts with the outside world: the head connects us to heaven; with our hands we contact each other by touching and by working together; the nipples are the contact that binds us with nourishment to the world; the genitals carry new life that can be born into the world; the anus connects us to the world through the cycle of matter, and the feet connect us to the earth through movement.

Other proverbs and ways of speaking also point to the fact that the feet embody the principle of movement. We talk of 'getting a foothold' and 'having a foot in the door', meaning that someone is on the way to achieving something. We say 'pull your socks up', meaning 'get going', and 'he has found his feet', meaning that he knows where he is going in life.

Although our feet carry us through life, they are a very neglected part of the body. Tight, ill-fitting shoes and insufficient freedom often cause great damage to the feet, and this obviously affects the reflex zones. There is a wide range of internal and external factors that affects the feet, which may or may not lead to disturbances in the referral zones, depending on the severity and duration of the irritation.

Common foot complaints can have the following causes:

1. Constant over-exertion and fatigue.
2. Injuries.
3. Inherited conditions (e.g. flat feet).
4. Circulatory problems (e.g. varicose veins).
5. Rheumatoid diseases.

Typical formations of the foot

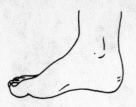
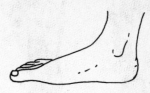

normal foot

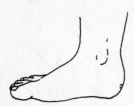
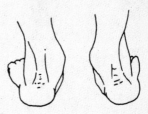

flat foot

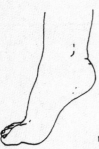
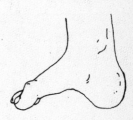

flat foot with pes valgus

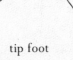

tip foot
talipes equinus

hollow foot

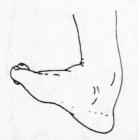
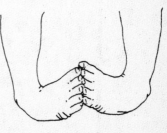

club foot
talipes calcaneo-valgus

club feet (talipeo
equinovarus)

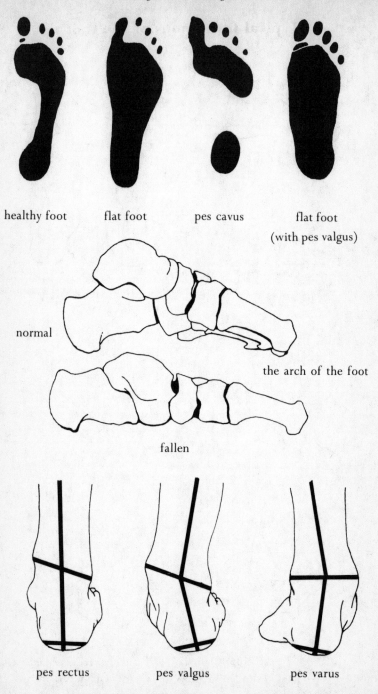

healthy foot   flat foot   pes cavus   flat foot
                                                      (with pes valgus)

normal

the arch of the foot

fallen

pes rectus   pes valgus   pes varus

Problems of these kinds always weaken the patient's general condition and may also point to specific disorders that may be treated with reflexology, although it is impossible to predict exactly what these might be or their duration. The practitioner is not in a position to make diagnoses, only to give therapy, though of course through treatment he will gain a clearer idea of the nature of the patient's complaint.

Build-up of pressure in the reflex zones detected by the therapist's hand or eye, or declared by a painfall reaction from the patient, may be caused by any of the following:

1. Over-exertion or over-tiredness.
2. Latent disease, whose symptoms are not yet evident.
3. Acute or chronic disease.
4. Hyperactive or deficient organ functioning.
5. Degeneration or atrophy.
6. Individual predisposition to disease (inherited tendency).
7. Injuries or accidents.

As we have already said, the practitioner should not try to make diagnoses—this is not the object of reflexology. To the patient's questions about the meaning of this or that pain, the therapist can answer that they are solely indications of disturbances in referral zones in the body. He can say which organs or parts of the body are affected, but exactly how and to what extent, he cannot tell.

Subjective experience/objective effects

The patient needs to be told what is about to happen before the massage begins. A short explanation of what reflexology is and what it sets out to achieve, its potential and its limitations, is essential at the outset. The patient should be told about his possible reactions to the massage so that he is prepared and has no false expectations or misconceptions about it. When the patient senses something happening in his body as a result of the massage, it means that the healthy process has begun and that his body has begun to mobilize its healing powers. When parts of the body that were rigid and tense are loosened through massage, this will also cause a corresponding loosening of the spirit, because reflexology works on the whole person, not just on his body, and it is not just the body that becomes charged with life, but the spirit too. Where there is movement, there is life, and where there is life, there is change. In this case we are not just talking about changing symptoms of disease, but changing the whole person.

The three basic activities of life are thought, action and movement. Together these realms form one unity. If there are inhibitions or blockages in one realm, this will clearly affect the other realms too. If we are working with reflex zone massage of the feet, we are dealing with the principle of movement, but there may also be changes in the realm of personality; there may be noticeable differences in the way a person thinks and acts.

Just as the therapy is not fixed and universally applicable in the same form, but is infinitely adaptable to each person and his own individual set of problems, there is no fixed set of reactions that the patient is bound to experience. The only thing that can be said to be universal is that all disturbed zones are extremely sensitive.

The therapeutic pressure of the thumb is often experienced as a sharp pricking pain, and right at the beginning of the treatment the patient can feel as if the therapist is sticking his thumb-nail deep into the foot. The patient's sensitivity to pain is an important guide for the rest of the treatment for that session, both in terms of duration and intensity of pressure.

We will differentiate between two types of reaction:
1. During treatments.
2. Between treatments.

1. Reactions during treatment can be audibly expressed by, for example, sighing or groaning, or they can be gestures of uneasiness or tensings of the muscles. The palms of the hands may begin to sweat, as may other parts of the body. This is an indication that the patient is reaching the limit of toleration to that particular phase of treatment. It should not be interpreted by the therapist as a sign that the massage has begun to 'work', as is so often thought. It means he should not push further in that particular area. If he continues, the next stage is a feeling of coldness that spreads from the patient's feet all the way up his legs. This cold sensation means that the transmission of energy has ceased to function and that the patient's tolerance of the treatment has already been over-extended.

Many therapists report tetanus-like cramps that can lead to circulatory problems (Marquandt, 1981). We have not observed these reactions, which anyhow indicate that the massage has been continued beyond the bounds of normal tolerance.

If the patient has any of the above-mentioned unpleasant reactions, the practitioner must alter his therapy accordingly to help normalize the disturbance. On no account should the treatment be broken off, but duration and intensity of pressure should be modified.

He should also use the technique already described, of alternating probing thumb massage with regular stroking movements, which give the body a chance to recover from the probing. If this method is followed the patient should get no more unpleasant reactions than a mild sweating of the palms.

After the massage the feet should feel relaxed and neither too warm nor too cool. After the first few sessions at the beginning of a course of treatment the body will not yet have developed its own heat regulator and, until it has, it may be necessary to warm the feet artificially with a blanket or hot-water bottle. The feet should not be left cold after a massage.

One sign that the patient is relaxed after a massage is that the joints at the base of the toes will feel loosened and supple to the therapist. The cracking of joints that often accompanies the 'lifting' of the toes from the basal joints is one of several significant pointers to a generally relaxed body state. Another most important sign is the relaxing of the shoulder girdle, which will have been brought about by massaging the reflective zone.

2. The reactions between treatments give evidence of the effects of massage and are most noticeable between the third and seventh massage. If the treatments are regulated properly and carried out in a professional manner, these reactions should be seen as normal. They are signs that the body has begun to react, in a possibly painful or unpleasant way, as part of the healing process. Sufferers of chronic diseases tend to experience more pain and increased weakness at this time, because the disease has to be made acute before it can be completely healed.

According to the severity of the reaction, treatment can be regulated or postponed until the body has had the opportunity to work through the next stage of therapy.

The following reactions can occur between treatments:

1. The skin can be affected by the metabolic changes in the body. Increased sweating and pimples may result.
2. The kidneys can be stimulated into producing more urine. The patient may experience increased urination.
3. Improved skin tone and texture of tissue, due to improved circulation.
4. The patient may sleep much better, but good nights may be punctuated by some nights of restlessness.

5. Regular and more frequent bowel movements, often accompanied by wind.

6. Increased secretion of the mucuous membranes in the nose, mouth and bronchials.

7. Short bouts of feverishness. Fever is one of the body's natural defences and it should not be suppressed. In this case, it is not a sign of illness.

8. Latent illnesses may appear. Often an illness that has been suppressed or has not been completely cured may be reactivated by the massage and eventually cured this way.

9. Psychic changes and alteration of attitude. Not infrequently a change in the patient's basic mood or humour is brought about by this holistic method of treatment. This is often associated with changes of attitude that can affect the patient's whole way of life. Patients may also often laugh or weep during treatments.

If the therapist is working together with a doctor, an evaluation of the patient's reaction should not prove problematical. A doctor should in any case be consulted if the therapist suspects a serious illness, and the patient should be encouraged to consult his own doctor.

To be a master in your subject, you must know its limits. Reflex zone massage has great potential, but it also has its limits. The more we understand and accept its limitations, the more we can hope to achieve for our patients.

Reactions of the therapist

The therapist is also prone to experience certain reactions because of the circulation of energy between himself and the patient. It is useful to know what these might be in order to prepare yourself. Often it is simply a feeling of tiredness accompanied by a compulsion to yawn; more rarely, there can be feelings of nausea and headache, but these are always preceded by warning symptoms, so preventative action can be taken. Amongst these symptoms are hot or cold throbbing fingers. This symptom can be cured by shaking the hands vigorously downwards or holding them under cold running water, a procedure that should be followed in any case at the end of a massage session. Yawning, coughing or sighing should not be suppressed—they are all signs that the body is freeing itself of disturbed energy. It is sensible to tell the patient about this, in case he misinterprets your yawning.

Measures to take in the case of unexpectedly strong reactions

It is possible that despite all precautions and carefully gauged treatment a patient may show unexpectedly strong reactions. In this case, proceed as follows. The first thing is to remain calm and observant: your main object should be to calm the patient. Bear in mind the Arndt-Schulz rule, which states that 'weak stimuli are beneficial, strong stimuli are detrimental, and very strong stimuli are harmful'. We can deduce from this that the patient has been over-stimulated and thrown off balance by the strength of his reaction. Very gentle stimuli will be necessary to restore the patient's balance.

If the patient shows signs of uneasiness during the massage, gentle stroking movements on both feet are often enough to calm him. To stretch and relax the pelvis, open the chest and ease breathing where the diaphragm is tense, the three-dimensional heel-grip illustrated in the colour plate section is very effective. Gentle stimulation of the zones of the solar plexus on both feet simultaneously, will lead to relaxation of the diaphragm and a general feeling of harmony. If necessary, the endocrine glands can be stimulated by gentle massage of the zones of the pituitary, parathyroid and adrenal glands.

If signs of an 'emergency' of this sort arise, the therapist will find that it often suffices to interrupt the massage and enfold the patient's feet in his hands, to give a sense of warmth and security and of being 'in safe hands'. This often dispels the fear of unexpected reactions. The patient can also be left undisturbed (though under observation) for a while to recover himself. If necessary, he should be kept warm with blankets.

It should also be mentioned here that gall stones and kidney stones may begin to move as a result of zone massage, which will facilitate movement of any deposits or blockages in the system. Should this happen, or be suspected, the therapist should work in conjunction with a doctor and encourage the patient to seek a consultation.

The question of the patient's age

You may wonder whether a patient is too young or too old for this type of treatment but, as reflex zone massage is concerned fundamentally with the patient rather than with illness, and with the patient's feelings rather than with his symptoms, age is not important. Restrictions on treatment are naturally determined by the individual's threshold of pain and his reactions to the massage. As long as the patient's body is able to cope with and respond to the stimulation of massage, there can be no qualms about its application. It is also to be recommended to elderly people who have no specific complaint—they will benefit from a couple of courses of treatment a year to tone up their body functions and give them a generally improved sense of well-being.

We have also had good results with the treatment of children, and even with babies. Most children are more relaxed and supple than adults and actively enjoy a gentle and correctly gauged reflex zone massage. Therapy often has unexpectedly swift results with child patients. Their young bodies are highly receptive to therapeutic stimuli. The older the patient and the longer he has been subjected to the various disturbances in his body, the more manifest those disturbances will be, and they will take a corresponding amount of time and effort to heal.

It is also comparatively easy to treat inherited complaints in children, who show a swifter response than their parents!

Length of treatment/number of sessions

If the patient is not suffering from an acute disorder, two courses of treatment a year will revitalize and stabilize his energy. When there are acute problems, the massage lasts for about 10 minutes and should be given daily at the beginning of the treatment. In the absence of acute problems, it is difficult to predict how many sessions each individual will need. This depends on several factors.

1. The patient's constitution.
2. The history of his illness.
3. His age.
4. The ability of his body to react to treatments.
5. His way of life.
6. His attitude to the treatment.

Basically, as long as the patient continues to react positively to treatment, it is worthwhile pursuing it. In general, a course of treatment will consist of between eight and twelve massage sessions. We would recommend two sessions a week for the first couple of weeks, and one session a week after that. This does not take into account the manifestation of acute disturbances or strongly adverse reactions, which the experienced therapist will know how to deal with as a matter of urgency.

Quite often, the patient will show a dramatic improvement after only one session. Subsequent sessions will then serve to stabilize his condition and consolidate his improvement.

The first session—the personal encounter with the patient and the physical and visual examination—will take about twice as long as subsequent sessions. The average session takes about 25 minutes for the massage. There is a danger of 'overdosing' the patient if the massage goes on for too long, and if it is too short, insufficient therapeutic stimulus will be provided for the body to be able to mobilize its own healing powers.

If there is still no reaction after several sessions, the body is probably temporarily unreceptive to therapeutic stimuli, and it may be advisable to break off the treatment for a while to give it a chance to adjust. There may also be external factors blocking the therapeutic impulse; for example, the patient may be heavily reliant on medication. If so, the situation can be discussed with the patient's doctor. It is possible that though no physical changes may be apparent, progress may be taking place on another level, perhaps in the patient's psychological attitude to life. This kind of change often results from the patient's awakened sense of his own body, which is one of the gifts of zone therapy. A change of this nature, which occurs in the patient's consciousness, will also gradually manifest itself in his body, given enough time.

Self-treatment and mechanical aids

Self-treatment is an important and necessary complement to any successful form of therapy or medical treatment. It is also important as an acknowledgement of responsibility for one's own health. Looked at from this angle, there is in principle nothing wrong with self-treatment.

If there are no acute problems, massaging one's own feet is a very useful way of instilling a general feeling of well-being, improving the circulation in the feet and the supply of blood to the various reflex zones. However, the following points about self-treatment should be borne in mind:

1. It is impossible to achieve the degree of relaxation so important to a patient.
2. The therapeutic impulse cannot be maintained at a constant because the body is both giving and receiving.
3. The influence exerted by the personality of the therapist is absent, and there is no harmonizing exchange of energies.
4. It is difficult, and sometimes impossible, to perceive one's own bodily reactions.

5. The hands quickly get tired because of the uncomfortable position.

6. Because of the above problems, there is a significantly reduced chance of success. Often no reaction is observed at all, in which case the patient/therapist may reject the whole idea of reflexology as unworkable.

There are many therapists who work with mechanical aids such as probes, rollers, spheres, mats, brushes and other gadgets. Anyone who uses these cannot be said to be acting in the true spirit of reflex zone massage. Gadgets get between the therapist and patient and rob the patient of the human contact so necessary for healing. The experienced and sensitive hand of the therapist cannot be replaced by an inert mechanical device.

Oils should not be used in reflex zone massage as they make the grip difficult to hold and the foot slippery to work with. The thumb would be constantly sliding out of position and the foot would not feel secure in the therapist's hands.

After the massage, the feet can be refreshed by rubbing with various oils or ointments if the patient wishes, but he should be advised against using foot sprays, as these clog the pores and prevent perspiration, which means that poisons the body needs to eliminate are kept inside.

The use of mechanical aids makes the value of massage very questionable. Mats and rollers may be harmless when used infrequently with patients who have no acute problems, but if the patient does have a disorder and mechanical aids are applied, nothing will be discovered about the deeper nature of the problem or its connections with other parts of the body, and because of ignorance, the treatment will probably do more harm than good.

Here is a case in point. A 45-year-old man had a foot roller under his desk at work, and used it constantly all the time he was there. After only a few days he collapsed and was taken to hospital. He underwent two weeks of very unpleasant examinations and at the end of it was surprised to learn from his doctors that there was nothing wrong with him. Extremely distressed, he came to see us. After four sessions his condition stabilized fully. Only on his fourth visit did he tell us about the gadget that he had bought and had been using so enthusiastically before his collapse—something that he had also neglected to tell the doctors. It was immediately obvious that the temporary but quite severe disorder that this man suffered could be attributed directly to his ignorance in treating himself with this so-called therapeutic gadget. This is a typical example of the trouble that can be caused by using this type of implement.

There is simply no substitute for the human hand in reflexology. The hand of the therapist is sensitive to the patient's needs and can gauge his treatment so as not to overstep them.

Unsuitable cases for treatment

As we have said, every form of therapy has its limitations and reflexology is no exception. It is important that these limitations should be recognized, and every reasonable practitioner should be ready to refer his patient elsewhere, should his own form of treatment prove inadequate in dealing with certain problems. People with the following conditions should not be treated with reflex zone massage:

1. Infectious diseases.
2. Acute fevers.
3. Inflammations of the venous system.
4. Inflammations of the lymphatic system.
5. Conditions requiring surgery.
6. Diseases of the foot that make treatment impossible.
7. Pregnancies which are at risk
8. Patients who are suffering from chronic depression or who are receiving heavy medication.

In cases of severe illness, such as cancer, multiple sclerosis or paralysis, reflexology cannot remove the cause of the disease, but it may significantly improve the patient's general condition because:

1. It can significantly relieve pain.
2. It can activate the excretory organs and stimulate the respiratory system.
3. It can help the patient achieve better control of the bladder and bowels.

To sum up

We have now explored the basic essentials of reflex zone massage. Before we turn to the particulars of the treatment itself, it may be useful to summarize the principles.

1. In the case of specific disorders it is always advisable to work as far as possible with a doctor, and preferably with a doctor who

is familiar with the concept and treatments of reflexology.

2. Reflex zone massage of the feet is one of a number of reflex zone therapies. Diagnosis is not its prime objective. It can, however, establish the existence of troublesome build-ups and disturbances in the reflex zones, and set about treating them. Above all, foot reflexology is an excellent method of preventative therapy.

3. When reflexology is used to treat a sick person, the principles of all holistic therapy apply. We are not treating an illness, but the person himself. We are concerned not with the symptoms, but with the underlying causes of the illness.

4. Reflex zone therapy should not be used indiscriminately. A responsible therapist will recognize both its potential and its limitations, and will realize that it is not an instant do-it-yourself panacea.

5. Although the hand concentrates on massaging a small part of the body—the feet—the therapist must never lose sight of the fact that he is treating the whole person.

6. Reflex zone massage is a natural method of healing and is compatible with all other natural healing methods, such as fasting to purify the body, hydrotherapy, homoeopathy, dietetic methods, deep breathing exercises, acupuncture, and aerobics. However, if more than one method is undertaken at one time, the patient should take care not to overdo it. If the body is bombarded with therapeutic stimuli, it may do more harm than good.

7. One good rule to abide by is that where there is over-activity, the therapist should bring calm, and where there is sluggishness, he should introduce stimulation.

8. There is no mechanical substitute for the skilled and sensitive hand of the responsible therapist.

9. The best qualifications a reflex zone therapist can have are a broad theoretical knowledge, an understanding of the interactions of body and soul, a positive inner attitude to the patient, a palpable, physical sense of the patient's well-being and a well-developed therapeutic integrity.

10. Reflex zone massage is a treatment in the literal sense of a 'handling'. The patient is literally 'handled', or treated with the hands.

11. Human contact and sensitivity are the most important criteria in any kind of therapy. All methods of healing that have a *person* as their focal point rely intensely on personal contact. The personal contact built up between reflexologist and patient is its

greatest asset. If reflex zone massage is used merely as a technique, a random mechanical prodding of various parts of the feet, we will have thrown away our greatest chance of success.

5

The Reflex Zones of the Feet

At the first treatment the zones will not be worked through with the usual degree of intensity, but they will be probed for any abnormalities. Abnormalities are detected by comparing the patient's reactions to a pressure of uniform intensity on the various zones. From the patient's sensitivity the therapist will be able to deduce which zones are normal and which, if any, are disturbed.

The preliminary investigation, the massage and its therapeutic results will all benefit from allowing the patient to have as much say in the matter as possible. In talking about his problems he will free himself of nervousness and inhibitions. The more calm and relaxed the patient is at the beginning of the session, the easier the therapist's work will be. In addition, the patient's account of what is troubling him will often give the first clues as to the cause of the disorders revealed by the therapist's examination.

What really distinguishes the experienced therapist is his ability to gauge the degree and extent of treatment needed. Success and failure largely depend on his judgement. The therapist should keep constantly in tune with his patient's reactions and make sure he does not push the patient too far, or overtax him.

The zones on the feet are easy to recognize once you have committed them to memory. As already mentioned, their relationship with each other corresponds to the anatomical structure of the body. Of course a knowledge of the zones will not guarantee success, as the student of reflexology will soon find out when he starts work. It should also be remembered that the position of the zones is liable to vary slightly with each individual.

It is important always to bear in mind that the zones themselves and the parts of the body they relate to are not the object of treatment—treatment always revolves around the whole person, and as often as not his problems are rooted, not in the zone where they appear to be located, but elsewhere. Holistic therapy mobilizes what Paracelsus called 'man's inner healer' and stimulates the body into healing itself. Once the body's own healing powers have been set in action, the therapist's job is to give them all the support they need to complete the body's recovery.

Holistic therapy sees man in terms of energy—healing powers and life forces. It is concerned with the forces flowing through the body which are the very essence of life itself. They determine personality and they determine physical characteristics too. In the circulation of the blood, in the lymphatic system and in the plasma in the cells, energy is constantly flowing through the body. The body's energies also interact with the natural and social world around it. We all react to our surroundings and, in this play of action and reaction, the body is the expression of the relationship between man and the world. Man does not have a body, he is a body, in which all the experiences of his life are stored. These experiences often take the form of tension in different parts of the body, and tension blocks the flow of energy through the system. Thus it is possible to understand how reflex zone therapy is actually a treatment of the experience of life translated into physical form. This is why 'symptoms' do not invariably point to certain isolated organic malfunctions, but are an expression for the situation in which the whole human organism finds itself, body and soul.

The organic reflex zones

The following list shows at a glance the various organic zones and their constituents.

1. *The zones of the musculo-skeletal system*
   spine, joints, musculature

2. *The zones of the head*

   skull
   temples
   sinuses
   jaw
   cerebrum
   cerebellum
   neck
   eyes
   ears
   teeth

nose and throat (tonsils, lymph glands, thyroid, parathyroid)

3. *The zones of the respiratory organs*
   mouth, nose, throat
   trachea, bronchials
   lungs, ribcage, diaphragm

4. *The zones of the digestive organs*
   mouth, oesophagus
   stomach, pancreas
   small intestine, colon, rectum
   gall bladder, liver
   appendix

5. *The zones of the heart*

6. *The zones of the urinary organs*
   kidneys, ureters
   bladder

7. *The zones of the lymphatic organs*
   upper lymphatics
   auxillary lymph nodes
   spleen, appendix
   lympathics of the groin
   lymphatics of the pelvis

8. *The zones of the endocrine glands*
   thyroid
   parathyroid
   adrenal glands
   pancreas
   ovaries, testes, prostate
   uterus (treated with the glands because of its functional
   connections)

Systematic representation of the reflex zones

The following gives a brief general description of the structure, situation and function of the organs and of the corresponding position of the reflex zones with reference to treatment. Throughout the book there are also references to the significance of disorders in these zones in a holistic context. These references are to be regarded as general background information, which may need to be adapted slightly each time it is applied.

Illness and its manifestations are, according to the holistic viewpoint, only the embodiment of the patient's prevalent condition. Thus backache may be a sign that the sufferer is weighed down by a heavy load (carrying his own cross). Another person may seek through illness the love and attention he is denied and craves so badly. In such a case, illness is a sort of refuge where the patient can get what he otherwise lacks in life. This kind of illness is mostly a hidden and quite unconscious call for help. Emotional problems find a corresponding expression of the body, in a person's bearing, voice and breathing.

All these things must be taken into account by the therapist in his consideration of the best way to help the patient. Perfectly healthy normal people exist only in textbooks. In reality sickness belongs to health, just as much as death belongs to life. Being ill is part of the imperfect and vulnerable business of being human, and it is most important that the patient should have an open and honest relationship with his body in sickness as well as in health.

The zones of the musculo-skeletal system

The Spine (*columna vertebralis/spina dorsalis*)
The spine is the backbone, the body's most important support, carrying the weight of the trunk. The spinal canal houses the spinal cord, the central channel of the nervous system running through the bone marrow. The spinal presents a double 'S' shape from the side view and consists of 34 or 35 vertebrae. These are:

 7 cervical vertebrae
12 thoracic vertebrae
 5 lumbar vertebrae
 5 sacral vertebrae
 4 or 5 coccycal vertebrae

The spine is an important axis of movement. It supports the shoulder girdle and the pelvic girdle and carries the free-moving skull. In the average adult human the spine is 75 cm (30 inches) long.

Tiny joints join each vertebrae to the next. The vertebrae get bigger lower down the spine, according to the increased weight they have to bear.

A *scoliosis* is a sideways curvature of the spine. It is usually, though not always, indicative of a malformation or disease of the spine. All the vertebrae are the same basic shape, with the exception of the first two cervical vertebrae (atlas and axis).

The mobility of the individual vertebrae is facilitated by the

Spine	No. of vertebrae	Shape	Name of curvature
neck	7	shallow backwards curve	cervical lordosis
chest	12	pushes forwards	thoracic kyphosis
loins	5	curves backwards	lumbar lordosis
sacrum	5*	points forwards	sacral and coccygeal kyphosis

coccyx the 4 'tail bones' of the spine are fused together to become one between the ages of 20 and 30

small discs (*disci invertebrales*) between them, which act as shock absorbers. When pressure is exerted on them they are compressed; when the pressure is released, they spring back to their normal shape. The discs are constantly being compressed and extended by the movements of the spine.

Pronounced sideways curvature of the spine causes a deformed chest cavity, which can in turn mean the displacement or distortion of the internal organs (heart and lungs).

The spine and intervertebral discs are subject to a certain amount of normal wear and tear. If this is excessive, bony growths can form on the edges of the vertebrae, causing a stiffening of the joints between them. As a result, pressure is exerted on the nerves running through the spinal column and the patient may suffer chronic backache and severely reduced flexibility of the spine. It has been shown that many patients with this kind of disorder (spondylosis, spondylarthrosis) benefit considerably from hydrotherapy, sun-lamp treatment and massage therapy of the reflex zones of the spine.

The reflex zones of the spine are found running along the inner side of both feet.

The reflex zones of the spine are massaged by applying pressure to the musculature of the feet in the relevant part. Massage on the ridge of the bone (*periosteum*) is important when treating the reflex

*the 5 sacral vertebrae are locked together. Men have a slightly longer sacrum with a more pronounced curve than women.

The spine

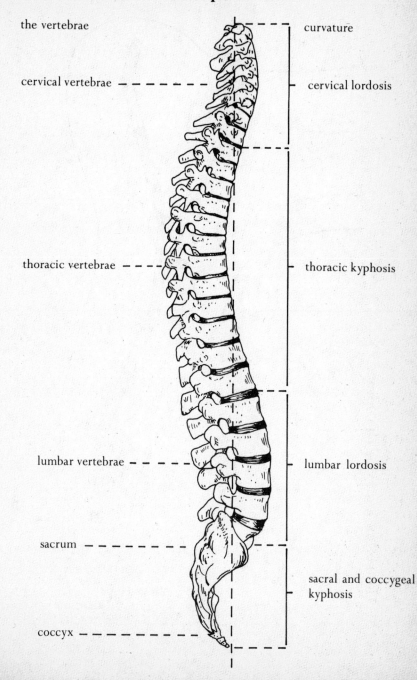

the vertebrae

cervical vertebrae

thoracic vertebrae

lumbar vertebrae

sacrum

coccyx

curvature

cervical lordosis

thoracic kyphosis

lumbar lordosis

sacral and coccygeal kyphosis

The reflex zones of the spine

right foot—inner aspect

The reflex zones of the spine are the same in both feet

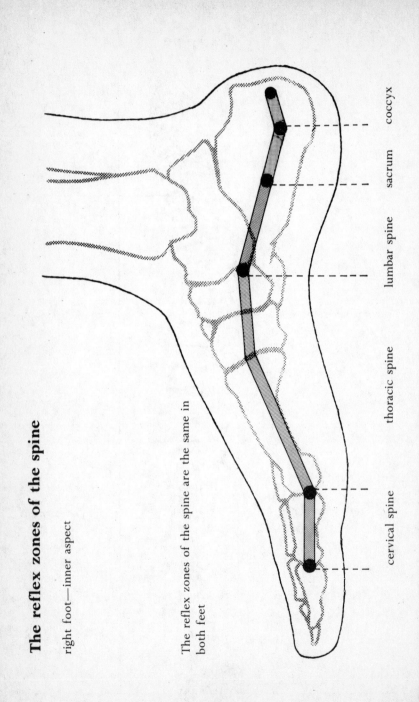

coccyx

sacrum

lumbar spine

thoracic spine

cervical spine

Referral zone	Position
cervical spine	medial aspect of the proximal phalanx of each big toe
thoracic spine	first metatarsal
lumbar spine	from the first cuneiform to the middle of the navicular
sacrum	from the proximal end of the navicular through the talus and into the calcaneum
coccyx	end of the calcaneum

zones of the nervous system, which should definitely be left to the experts.

Massage of the reflex zones of the spine is an important part of the treatment because of its ability to relax the patient, and for this reason it usually forms the first stage of a reflex zone massage.

In the reflex zone of the neck (the joint formed by the phalanx of the big toe and the first metatarsal) there is often a condition called hallux valgus (see the photograph in the colour plate section), where the big toe turns inwards towards the other toes. This is often a sign of a disorder in the neck, but because each area affects the other, it is often not possible to say which came first, the hallux valgus or the disorder in the neck. The majority of patients with complaints in the neck area show one or more of the following:

1. A distortion of the bones in the cervical spine.
2. Tension in the neck and shoulders.
3. Complications of the thyroid gland.

Relief of pain and a release of tension in the spine can be accomplished by a passifying massage, working through the zones of each part of the spine. Pressure should be exerted with the inner side of the end of the thumb for about 30 seconds each time.

Joints and musculature

It is man's mobility that enables him to react to his surroundings. If his mobility is limited, he will be less able to effect a change in his surroundings.

The bones and joints are the structural or passive part of the mobility system, and the muscles are the active part. They operate the joints and set the body in motion. The work of the muscles is co-ordinated by the nervous system.

The musculature of the body makes an important contribution to its shape. One of the main objectives when working on the mobility system is to relax the muscles, which will make the body more mobile, restore spontaneity of movement to the patient and make him feel more alive and more lively. In many cases where a patient's movement is impaired, exercise can do a great deal to improve both mobility and general health, and should be recommended.

The following areas are of prime importance in reflex zone massage of the feet:

1. Neck/shoulder girdle.
2. Shoulder joints.
3. Arms/elbows.
4. Rib-cage.
5. Abdomen/pelvis.
6. Hip joints/symphisis pubis.
7. Musculature of the buttocks.
8. Musculature of the upper thighs.

Massaging the reflex zone of the shoulder girdle (in the transverse arch across the five zones of each foot) is particularly effective with psychosomatic illness. Tension in the shoulders and neck is a sign of the burden a patient is 'shouldering' or the weight he is carrying 'round his neck'. Therapy is most successful on the dorsal side of the foot, where both muscular and nervous tension can be treated.

The zone corresponding to the shoulder joints will be felt at the basal joint of the little toes. One peculiarity arising from the division of the body into zones is that the zone of the upper arm down to the elbow is identical with that of the edge of the rib-cage nearest to it.

The zone relating to the musculature of the rib-cage extends across the metatarsals on both sides of the feet.

The muscles are connected to the nerves at motor end plates. Nervous signals are transmitted constantly through these, whether the muscles are in action or at rest. The constant transmission keeps the muscle in a state of readiness known as tonus. Tonus varies from individual to individual as well as from one group of muscles to the next, and can be weakened or

Reflex zones of the musculature of the body

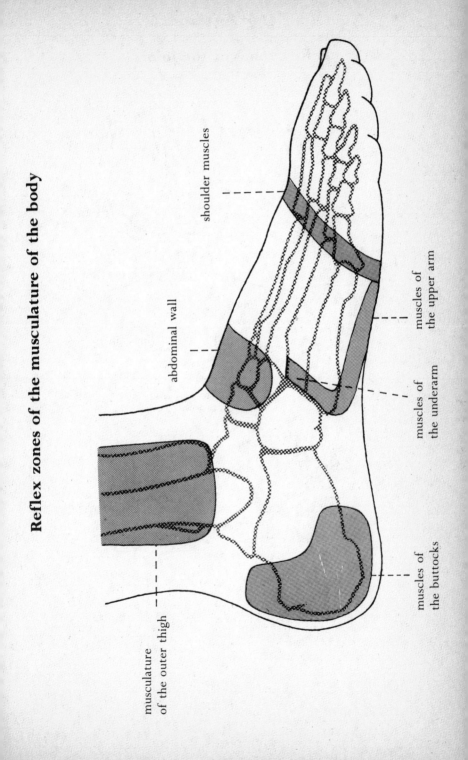

shoulder muscles

abdominal wall

muscles of the upper arm

muscles of the underarm

muscles of the buttocks

musculature of the outer thigh

Reflex zones of the joints

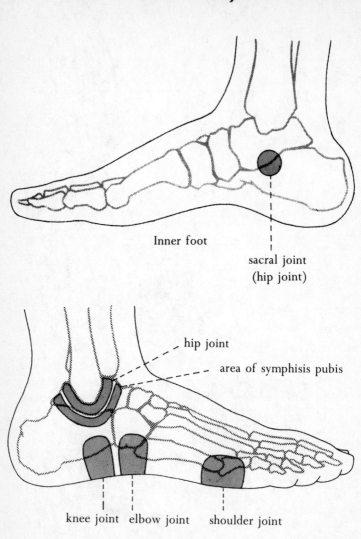

Inner foot

sacral joint
(hip joint)

hip joint

area of symphisis pubis

knee joint   elbow joint   shoulder joint

Outer foot

Reflex zones of the musculature

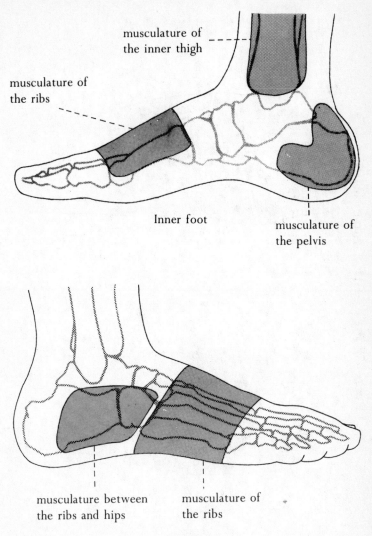

musculature of
the inner thigh

musculature of
the ribs

Inner foot

musculature of
the pelvis

musculature between
the ribs and hips

musculature of
the ribs

Outer foot

Reflex zones of the musculature

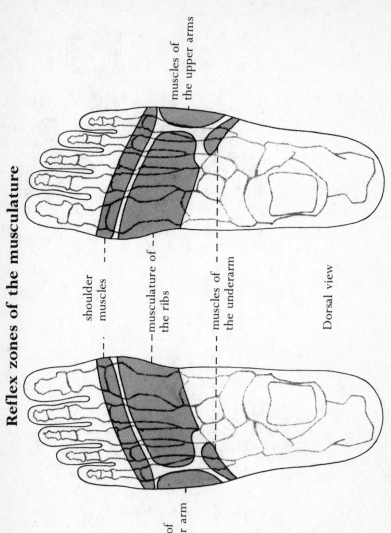

shoulder
muscles

musculature of
the ribs

muscles of
the underarm

muscles of
the upper arms

muscles of
the upper arm

Dorsal view

heightened by certain disorders of the nervous system. We can considerably improve muscle tonus with reflex zone massage.

What disorders of the musculo-skeletal system reveal about the patient

If we describe someone as being weighed down with work or responsibility, shouldering a heavy burden, or having a millstone around his neck or a chip on his shoulder, we are talking about constant psychological pressures which, if they persist, can manifest themselves in physical pain and changed bearing in exactly the areas referred to. Here again we see how important it is not to restrict our work to physical symptoms, but to look beyond them to their psychological or emotional causes.

If a person's muscles are tense when he is at rest, then we must deduce that certain emotions are being bitten back and suppressed, or aggressive impulses are being denied. The body is attempting to rid itself of these impulses through heightened muscle activity.

Though this muscle tension in a sense protects the sufferer from the things he fears, he will also fall victim to its erosive powers if the tension persists over a long period of time.

The zones of the head

Inside the skull are the brain, the sensory organs and the start of the respiratory and digestive tracts.

The reflex zones of the head are unusual in that they occupy all ten toes. They are also found replicated in miniature on both big toes.

Tension in the neck/head area can be relieved by exercising the joints of the big toe, as rotating the toe on its basal joint corresponds to rotating the head on the neck.

It has been shown that short-sightedness can be improved by treating the second toe, and long-sightedness by treating the third toe. The inner ear is represented by the fourth toe and the outer ear by the fifth toe. Eyes, ears and teeth are best treated from the sole and on the sides of the toes, but in general the zones of the head should be massaged from all sides.

Reflex zones of the head

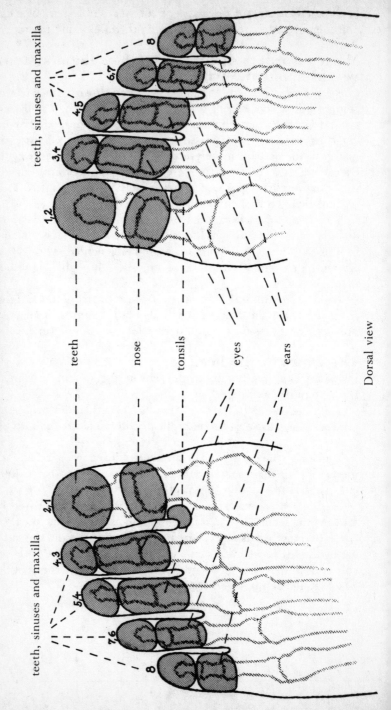

teeth, sinuses and maxilla

teeth, sinuses and maxilla

teeth

nose

tonsils

eyes

ears

Dorsal view

Reflex zones of the head

cerebrum ---
temporal lobe ---
mastoid process ---
neck ---

The soles of the feet

Reflex zones of the head

nose

jaw

mouth

upper
lymphatics

Dorsal view

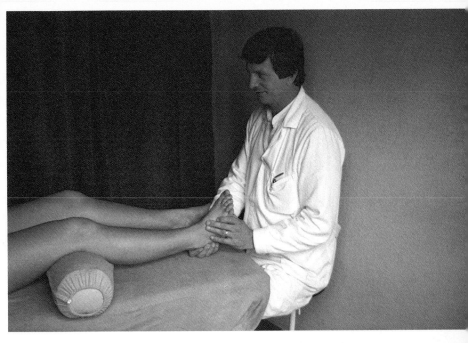

The patient should be relaxed and comfortable

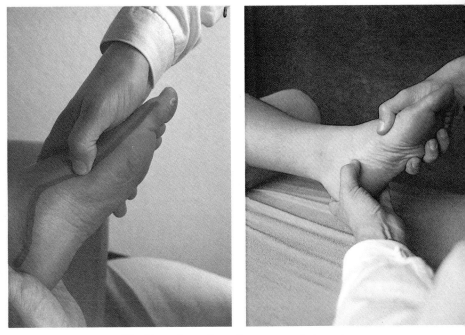

Working along the reflex zones of the spine

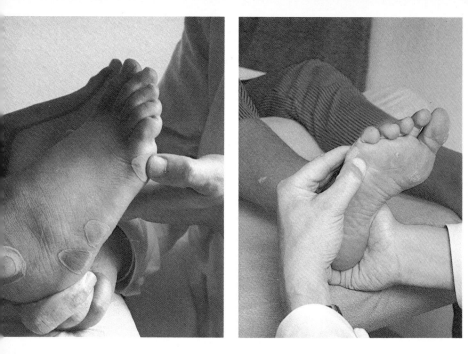

Working in the region of the shoulder joints

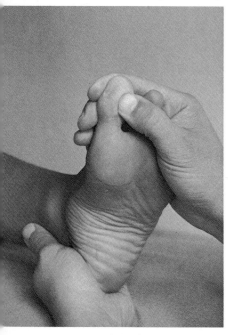

Massage of the head area
(pituitary)

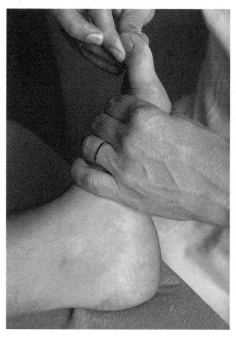

Manipulation of the big toe to
relax tension in the neck area

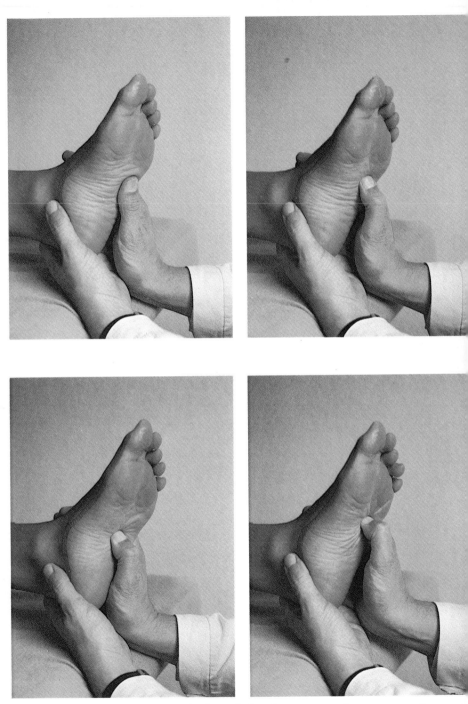

Progressive stages in a rhythmical thumb massage using pressure of
varying intensity

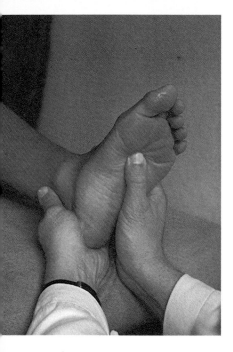
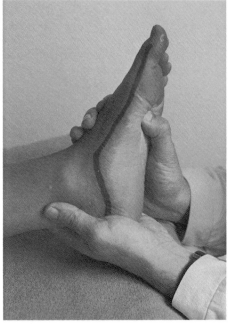

Relaxation exercise (solar plexus)

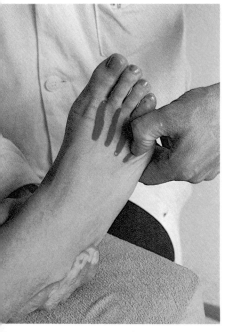

Stimulating the bronchials

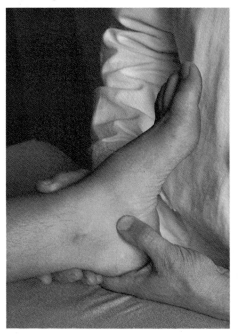

Lubricating the hip joint

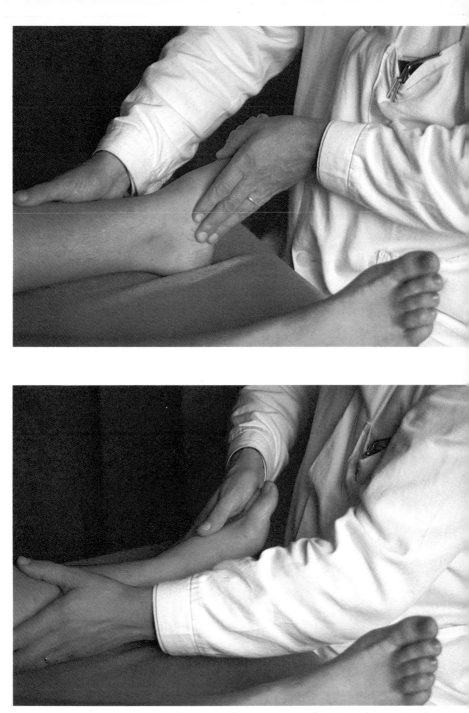

During massage use relaxing strokes: move your hands on the inside of the foot up towards the body, and on the outside of the foot towards the toes.

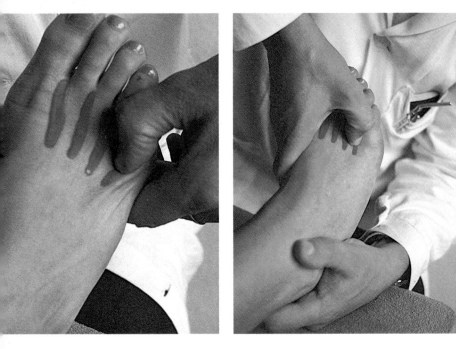

Grips for working on the bronchials

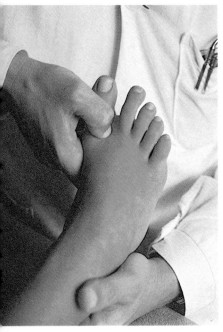

Massage in the area of the tonsils

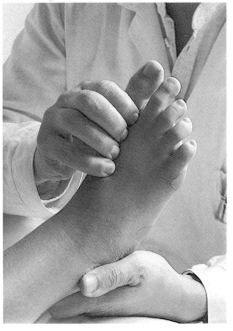

Frictional grip unblocking the lymph channels, working towards the toes

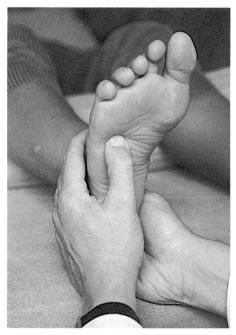

Grip for working on the gall
bladder

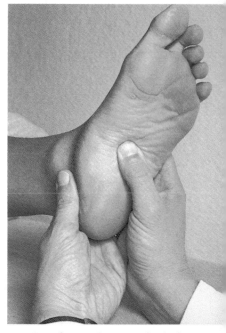

Grip for working on the kidneys

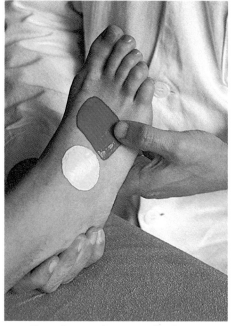

Grip for working on the lungs,
using the top of the foot

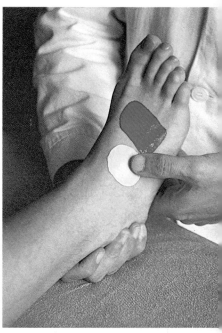

Grip for working on the musculature of the stomach

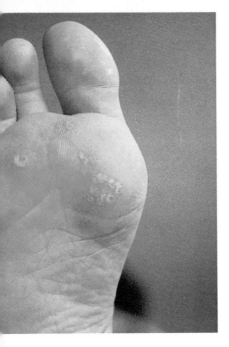

Warts in the thyroid reflex zone

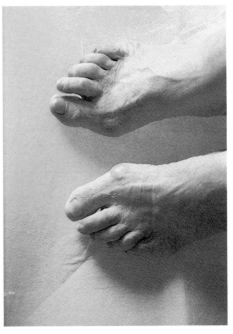

Hallux valgus

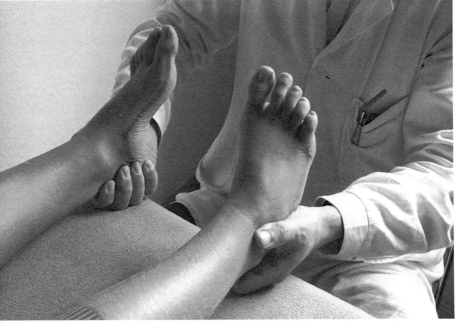

The three-dimensional grip on the heels releases tension in the respiratory system and the pelvis

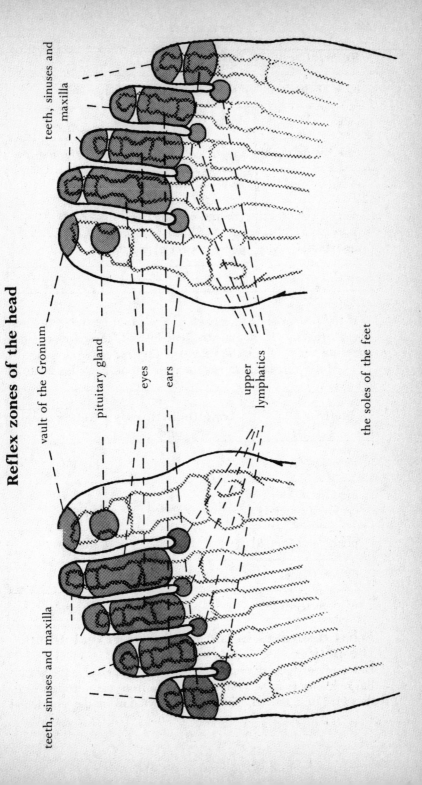

Reflex zones of the head

teeth, sinuses and maxilla

teeth, sinuses and maxilla

vault of the Cronium

pituitary gland

eyes

ears

upper lymphatics

the soles of the feet

Referral zone	Position
back of the head	ball of the big toe (plantar side)
face	dorsal side of big toe
base of the skull	the crease under the ball of the big toe
eyes	2nd and 3rd toes
ears	4th and 5th toes
nose/throat cavity	dorsal aspect of big toe
upper lymphatics	the webs of the toes

If the patient shows signs of athlete's foot between the toes, these areas should not be treated. Instead, the corresponding zones on the hands, in between the fingers, can be massaged.

The following chart shows the position of the reflex zones of the teeth:

Teeth	Longitudinal body zone	Reflex zone
incisors (1)	1	big toe
incisors and canines (2 and 3)	2	2nd toe
premolars (4 and 5)	3	3rd toe
molars (6 and 7)	4	4th toe
wisdom teeth (8)	5	5th toe

What disorders in the head area reveal about the patient

Here are our sensory organs, with which we perceive the world. But our sensory organs do not just take from the outside world, they give to it as well. The eye is our window on the world, and through it the world can see our feelings. The eye is the mirror of the soul, revealing the character and personality inside.

Short-sightedness and long-sightedness are the two most common eye problems. Short-sightedness is connected with youth and signifies egocentricity. Long-sightedness comes with old age and signifies objectivity and a better all-round view.

Problems with the eyes do not only mean that the patient can't see things; they often show that there are things he does not want to see. But though you can shut your eyes, your ears remain open. They represent a passive openness, a receptivity to the world. We say we are 'all ears', meaning we are receptive to information. The ear is often called 'impartial'. Hearing and listening are closely connected, though the first is passive and the second active. An unrelenting attitude and a stiff posture in old age often go hand in hand with being hard of hearing.

There are lots of sayings connected with the head. We say 'like bashing your head against a brick wall', 'so-and-so has completely turned his head', 'keep a cool head', 'hot-headed', 'it's gone to his head', and many other such phrases. Each has a particular meaning, and if only these meanings were taken seriously enough they could throw considerable light on some of the disorders of the head.

The head is one with the thought process, so that a headache is often a result of muddled thinking. The connection between the head and the lower body deserves particular consideration in cases of migraine. Dethlefsen and Dahlke write in their book *Krankheit als Weg* (The Path of Illness) that migraine is displaced sexuality manifesting itself in the head. The conflict is, as it were, taking place on a higher plane. It is a conflict between above and below, between head and genitals, and the head is the battle ground where the problem is thrashed out. It is a conflict that can only be truly solved if it is dealt with in its place of origin. The balance between above and below, between thought and action, should always be taken into account both with migraine and with headaches.

The zones of the respiratory tract

The respiratory tract, like the digestive tract, begins in the face, and the corresponding reflex zones on the foot therefore begin with the mouth and nose on the big toe.

The following table shows the location of the zones of the respiratory tract:

Referral zone	Position
mouth/nose cavity	big toe (dorsal aspect)
bronchials	laterally from the basal joint of the big toe towards the mid-point of the first and second metatarsals (plantar and dorsal)
lungs	all across the metatarsals
diaphragm	directly beneath the transverse arches

The diaphragm divides the respiratory system from the digestive system. The solar plexus bears the brunt of the conflict between the upper and lower halves of the body. In many people one half dominates the other. Work on the reflex zone of the diaphragm can therefore be most effective in establishing a balance. The diaphragm is the most important muscle for breathing. It is situated between the chest cavity and the abdomen. When the diaphragm contracts, it enlarges the chest cavity and breath is drawn in. As the diaphragm relaxes, it pushes up into the chest cavity and air is expelled from the lungs.

Although the diaphragm extends across the whole of the trunk, there is one small zone on the foot that is particularly effective in its treatment. It lies directly beneath the transverse arch in longitudinal zones 2 and 3. It is also the reflex zone of the solar plexus.

The sensitive treatment of the solar plexus is very important in reflexology: it can relieve stress and nervousness, aid deep regular

Patient's breathing	Therapeutic stimulation
inhaling	exert gentle pressure on the reflex zone of the diaphragm with a three-dimensional pull on the heel (see photograph in the colour plate section)
exhaling	release the pressure, returning to the original position

breathing and restore calm. Massage of this zone will make the patient relaxed and receptive to other therapeutic stimuli. When the respiratory rhythm of the patient is followed, the massage can be most effective, with a considerable reduction of pain.

This movement should be repeated 15–20 times on each foot. As well as the benefits described above, it is also excellent for dealing with breathing problems.

What respiratory complaints reveal about the patient

Breath means life. A creature that breathes is alive, and a living creature is a breathing one. Breath is a direct connection between the self and the world. If we say of someone 'it took his breath away' or 'he held his breath', then it signifies that there was a disturbance in that person's relationship with his surroundings, the outside world. Breathing is an exchange, a giving and taking, contracting and relaxing. We should be able to open ourselves to it so that breath streams through our whole body. We cannot shut ourselves off from breathing, because it is what gives us life.

Through the air that we breathe, we are connected to everything around us. The first breath taken by a new baby means that he is independent and free. Difficulties with breathing are often a clear sign of fear of independence and freedom. Only when we feel free can we breathe freely. Everyone who has breathing problems should ask himself what is preventing him from giving to and taking from the world around him.

Asthma is a common complaint amongst sufferers from respiratory illness. The asthmatic's problem is that he takes too much. He draws too much breath, does not want to give any of it back and must therefore struggle to get more of the air he so desperately needs. Asthmatics have no balance between give and take. The asthmatic cannot catch his breath because he is holding too much of it back inside himself. He is often top-heavy and domineering. He has a basically hostile attitude to life. He is always ready to strike up an argument with the people around him, always at crossed swords with life. But he is incapable of working out his aggression, because he is paralysed by lack of breath. This stifling reaction robs him of the chance of freeing himself, living out his aggression and breathing freely.

The zones of the digestive tract

The digestive organs are responsible for delivering nourishment to the body, so that it has the strength to maintain itself and to grow,

Reflex zones of the respiratory tract

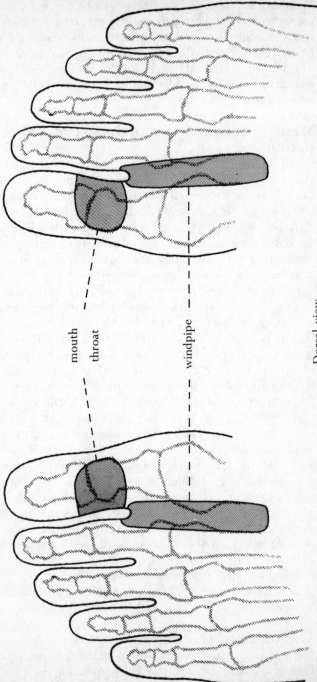

mouth
throat

windpipe

Dorsal view

Reflex zones of the respiratory tract

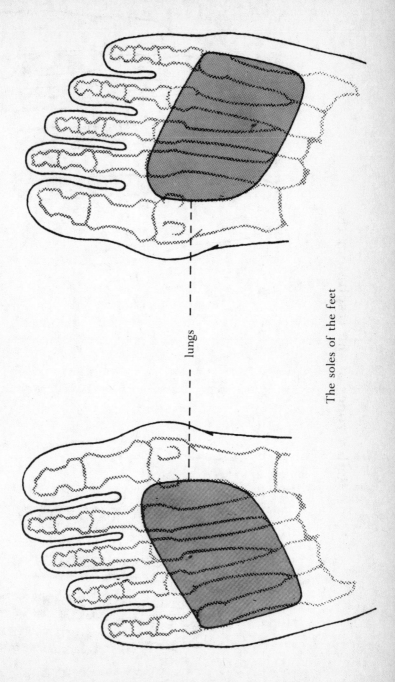

lungs

The soles of the feet

Reflex zones of the respiratory tract

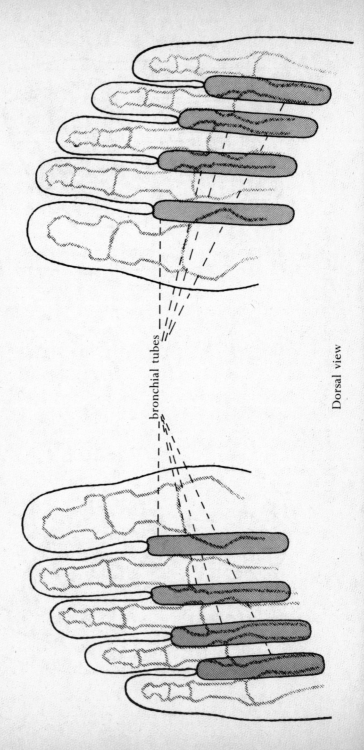

bronchial tubes

Dorsal view

Reflex zones of the respiratory tract

lungs

Dorsal view

Reflex zones of the respiratory tract

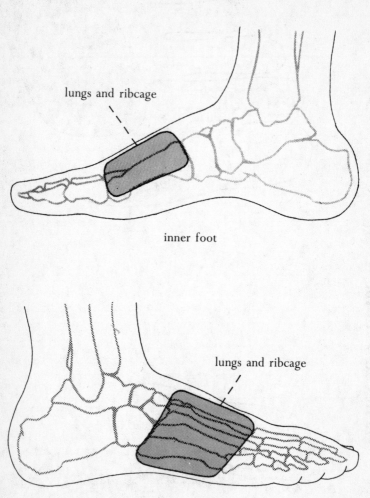

lungs and ribcage

inner foot

lungs and ribcage

outer foot

Reflex zones of the respiratory tract

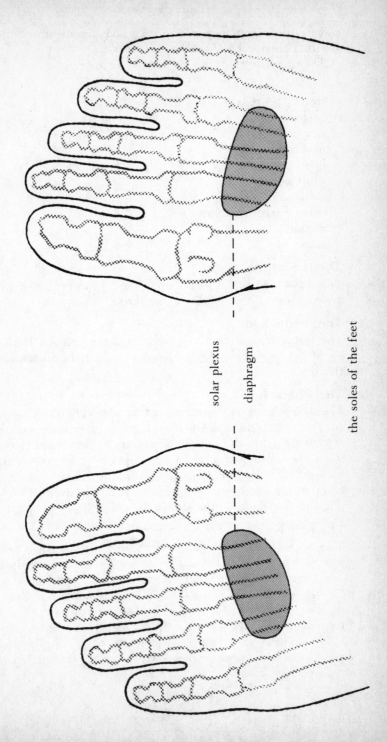

solar plexus

diaphragm

the soles of the feet

and also the energy required to keep body temperature constant and fuel chemical and mechanical activity.

The digestive tract can be divided as follows:

mouth, teeth
throat (pharynx)
oesophagus
stomach
pancreas
liver
gall bladder
small intestine
colon (large intestine)
rectum
anus

The throat (pharynx)

The throat consists of three parts. The respiratory and digestive systems join in the middle of the throat.

The oesophagus

The oesophagus connects the mouth with the stomach. It is a tube about 25 cm (10 inches) long, situated between the bronchials and the spine.

The stomach

The stomach lies on the left side of the upper abdomen, between the liver and the spleen. Behind it is the pancreas, which represents a broadening of the digestive tract. Peristalsis, the wave-like movement of the whole digestive tract, is controlled automatically by nerves in the stomach wall. Depending on composition and digestibility, food remains on average between one and five hours in the stomach.

The pancreas

This organ lies behind the stomach and is responsible for the production of digestive juices—between ½ litre and 1½ litres per day. Digestive juices contain enzymes capable of breaking down fat, protein and carbohydrate. The pancreas can be subject to inflammation (acute inflammation often strikes suddenly after a too-rich meal) and swelling. If the pancreas is removed, its function must be replaced by injection of insulin or enzyme tablets to avoid serious problems with blood sugar levels as well as with the digestion.

The liver

The liver is connected to the intestine and situated in the right upper abdomen, though it extends quite a way to the left. The liver fulfils an important metabolic function and is closely connected with the circulatory system. The functions of the liver are:

1. Glandular (produces bile).
2. Responsible for circulation of bilirubin (jaundice occurs when this function is impaired).
3. Metabolic (conversion of carbohydrates and other foods to glycogen, production of urea/detoxification).
4. Circulatory (manufacture of blood proteins and factors necessary for blood clotting).
5. Manufacture of iron-binding factors.

The small intestine

The small intestine is about 6 metres (20 feet) long, and is one of the most important sections of the digestive tract. It is here that nutrients are broken down into their simplest components for absorption by the epithelium, the wall of the intestine. The small intestine consists of the duodenum, jejunum and ileum. The movements of the intestine are autonomic, (that is, they are controlled by the nerves in the musculature). The contents of the small intestine are pushed in wave-like movements into the colon. Where the small intestine joins the colon there are two folds that act like valves, stopping the contents of the intestines from travelling backwards.

The colon

The colon surrounds the small intestine like a frame and can be divided as follows: caecum, ascending colon, transverse colon, descending colon, sigmoid colon. The process of digestion continues in the colon and terminates in the anus, an opening controlled by two muscles. The mucous membranes in the anal canal are deeply ridged and run through with veins. Haemorrhoids or piles is the condition that results when these veins swell abnormally.

What disorders in the digestive tract reveal about the patient

First let us look at a few more common phrases and sayings: 'a bad taste in the mouth', 'a lot to swallow', 'couldn't digest it all', 'makes the gorge rise', 'eaten up with something', 'to bellyache', '

Reflex zones of the digestive tract

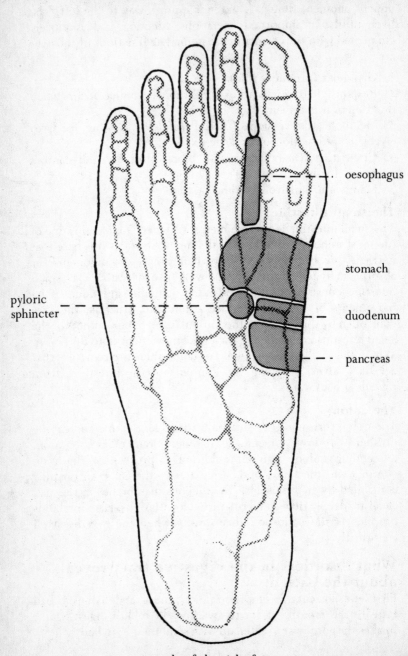

oesophagus

stomach

pyloric
sphincter

duodenum

pancreas

sole of the right foot

Reflex zones of the digestive tract

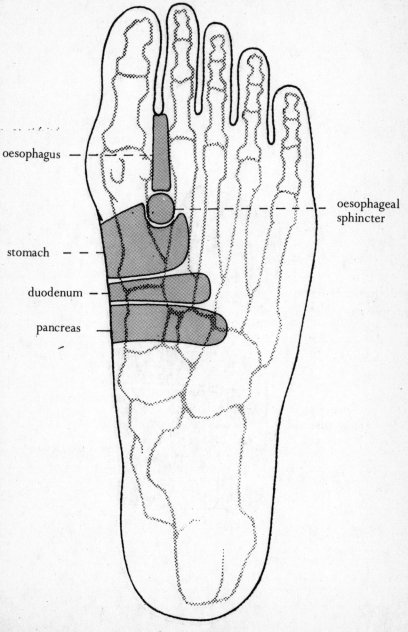

oesophagus

oesophageal
sphincter

stomach

duodenum

pancreas

sole of the left foot

Reflex zones of the digestive tract

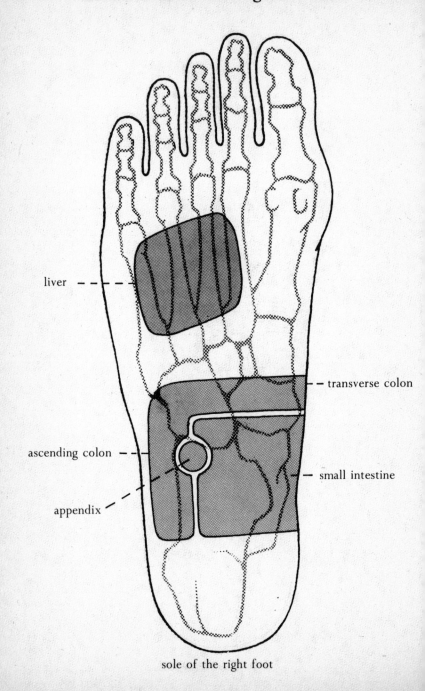

sole of the right foot

Reflex zones of the digestive tract

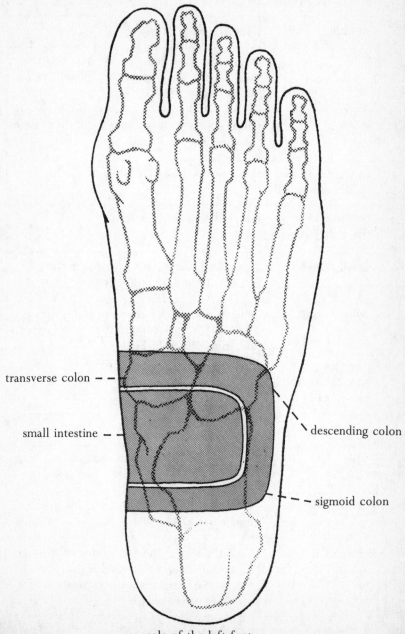

transverse colon – –

small intestine –

descending colon

sigmoid colon

sole of the left foot

'a consuming passion' and finally, 'the way to the heart is through the stomach'.

Referral zones	Position
mouth	dorsal aspect of big toe
throat/ oesophagus	from the basal joint of the big toe half way across the metatarsals (plantar and dorsal aspects)
stomach	on the soles of both feet around the base of the first metatarsal
cardia (entrance to the stomach)	treated on the left foot
pylorus (exit from the stomach)	treated on the right foot
small intestine	from Lisfranc's joint line downwards. Lateral boundary is longitudinal zone 4
colon	corresponds to its anatomical position as a 'frame' for the small intestine (see diagrams on pages 96 and 97)
sigmoid/rectum/ anal/area	on the soles of both feet in the area of the calcaneum and talus
pancreas	in the same zone as the stomach
liver	on the sole of the right foot in the metatarsals, longitudinal zones 2–5
gall bladder	on the top of the right foot, longitudinal zones 3 and 4
caecum and appendix	accessible from the dorsal side of the right foot, it is situated about 1.5 cm (½ inch) below the base of the metatarsals in longitudinal zone 5

The digestive system, like the respiratory system, is concerned with taking in substances from the outside world. These substances must be processed. Work starts with the teeth, and the teeth have always been a symbol of strength and vitality. After chewing comes swallowing. If someone has trouble in swallowing, he should ask himself whether there is something going on in his life that he cannot or does not want to swallow. It is then the stomach's turn to receive the food to be digested. It must be open and ready to receive it. This is a passive function.

The stomach's active function is the production of acids. If someone is unable to translate his anger into aggression and must swallow his anger, or bite it back, then the suppressed aggression activates the acids in the stomach. If normal aggression is not given an outlet but constantly turned inwards, the build-up of aggression can eventually cause stomach ulcers. A stomach ulcer is a sign that the stomach has begun, as it were, to digest itself, and the patient is being consumed with anger in the truest sense of the word. In this case, the patient should ask himself: 'What makes me sour? What makes me so acid? What is eating me up?' The answers to these questions should locate the conflict within him.

The small intestine is often compared to the brain, not only because of its visual similarity. The brain digests intangible matter, the intestine digests tangible matter. Diarrhoea is a sign of anxiety, and anxiety has mainly to do with a feeling of being constricted or restricted in some way. Diarrhoea shows the antidote to anxiety: it is an opening up and a letting go, a freeing of constriction.

The most common complaint of the colon is constipation. Constipation is symbolic of clamming up and holding on tight. This is associated with greed and a strong materialistic streak. Psychoanalysis interprets constipation as a fear of discovering the unknown.

The liver both delivers energy and takes away poisons. The first job here is to differentiate between what is poisonous and what is not. Disorders of the liver are sometimes a sign that the sufferer is having difficulty judging and evaluating things correctly. He does not know, for example, his own levels of tolerance. This is why the diseases of the liver are caused by excess: too much fat, too much alcohol. The liver reacts to overdoing things and a lack of moderation.

Permanent blockages lead to a damming up of energy, which

Reflex Zone Massage

Reflex zones of the digestive tract

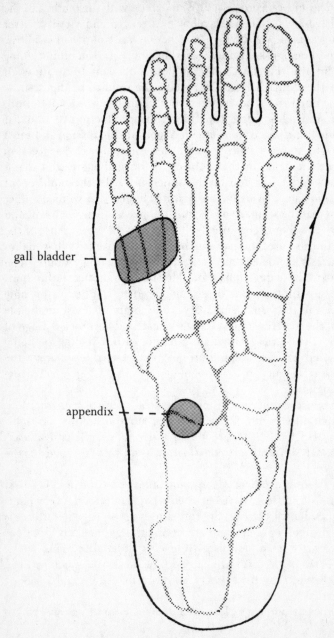

gall bladder

appendix

sole of the right foot

Reflex zones of the digestive tract

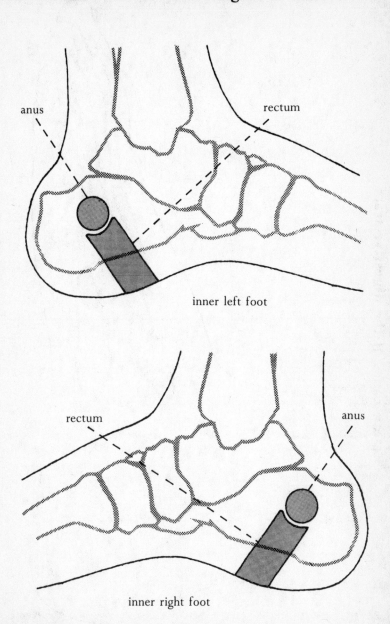

anus

rectum

inner left foot

rectum

anus

inner right foot

Reflex zones of the digestive tract

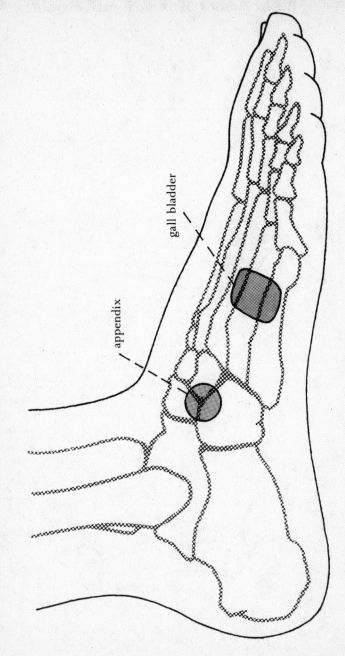

gall bladder

appendix

outer right foot

Reflex zones of the digestive tract

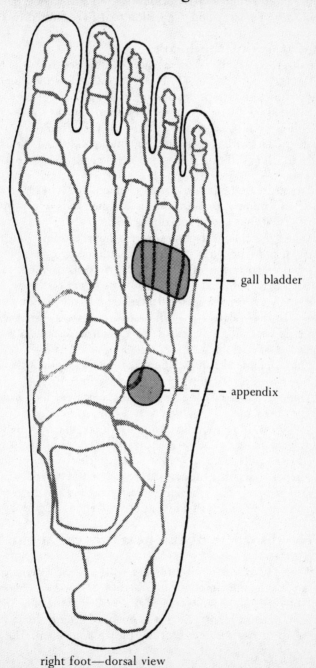

gall bladder

appendix

right foot—dorsal view

will show itself sooner or later in material form, such as the so-called stones found in the kidneys and gall bladder. These are build-ups of energy and aggression that have turned to stone.

The zones of the heart

We often say 'at the heart' meaning 'at the centre'—the heart is at the centre of the human body. It is a hollow muscular organ whose function is to pump blood through the circulatory system. The direction of the flow of blood is determined by valves. There is a dividing wall between the left and right sides of the heart. The left half deals with ciculation through the body, and the right half with the lungs. Both halves are divided into an auricle and a ventricle.

The heart is about as big as a clenched fist. It beats on average 70 times a minute, or 100,000 times a day, and pumps almost 7.5 litres (13¼ pints) of blood through the body.

When the therapist comes to treating the reflex zones of the heart, it is particularly important that he should free himself of the symptomatic way of thinking and view his partner as a whole person. It is comparatively rare for disorders of the heart to be caused by an organic disturbance there. They are much more likely to be related to functional disorders, whether of a psychological or a physical nature, such as problems with the digestion or breathing.

The principle to follow when treating the zones of the heart is 'depress hyperexcitability and stimulate flaccidity'.

The heart and the blood are symbols of life. Blood pressure is the result of the play between the flow of blood and its limits. Both high and low blood pressure can be regulated with a simple grip, stroking down both feet towards the toes in the furrows of the metatarsals with a gentle pincer grip of the thumb and forefinger. The same process can be carried out on the hands, the pincer grip moving from the wrist towards the fingers. Each movement, on feet or hands, should be carried out 10–20 times.

What disorders of the heart reveal about the patient

Someone with low blood pressure will avoid situations that call for a considerable amount of resistance or effort. Someone with high blood pressure is always under pressure. If the blood pressure rises momentarily, it releases a burst of energy for a specific purpose, to rise to a conflict or resolve a problem. The person

Reflex zones of the heart

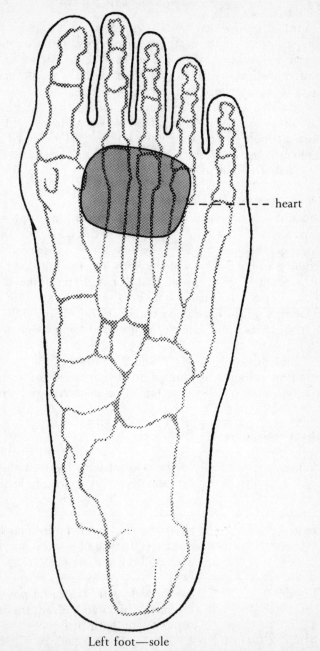

heart

Left foot—sole

with constantly high blood pressure will avoid solution by conflict, thus making it impossible to diffuse his energy in a productive way.

Turns of phrase that revolve around the heart cover a wide range of emotions: 'the heart bursts with joy', 'to take something to heart', 'broken-hearted'. The heart is a symbol of love, emotion and purity. It reacts spontaneously to all kinds of situations by a change in the rate of the heartbeat. When the heartbeat alters, this is sometimes the first sign that something out of the ordinary has happened, and it is a signal that should not be ignored. People with heart trouble fear being alone, and if people who live alone have heart trouble, it can be a sign that they long to be looked after and to be loved.

The zones of the urinary tract

The kidneys are a pair of 10–12 cm (4–5 inch) long bow-shaped organs whose axes do not run parallel to the spine, but converge above and behind it. The position of the kidneys changes according to the position of the body and the breathing.

The adrenals are the glands that lie next to the kidneys, which is how they get their name (kidneys = renes). Next to the lungs, the kidneys are the most important excretory organs in the body. The right kidney lies beneath the liver and the left one lies half-under the spleen.

In the course of one day about 1,500 litres (330 gallons) of blood flow through the kidneys. In the same space of time about three times the whole body fluid is filtered through them.

Referral zone	Position
kidneys	on the soles of both feet just above Lisfranc's joint line in longitudinal zones 2 and 3
ureters	along the tendon of the hallucis longis muscle (this tendon is easily located by bending back the big toe)
bladder	corresponds with its central position in the body—situated beneath the inner malleolus on both feet

One of the main tasks of the kidneys is to eliminate waste substances like urea and uric acid from the body. If the kidneys are not functioning properly, these substances get into the bloodstream. The kidneys also excrete water, salts and acids. Thus a malfunction of the kidneys can results in dropsy or an imbalance in the blood levels of sodium and potassium.

The ureters are tubes which take the urine from the kidneys to the bladder, which lies in the pubic area of the pelvis. The flow of urine from the bladder is checked by two muscles at its opening, which are essentially sensitive to reflex zone massage.

When treating the organs of the urinary tract it does not matter whether the massage proceeds from the kidneys to the bladder or vice versa, as urine is not only driven from the kidneys, but is also actively drawn towards the bladder.

Reflex zone massage of the adrenal glands has proved most effective in the treatment of all kinds of allergies.

What complications in the urinary tract reveal about the patient

In holistic terms, the kidneys symbolize partnership. Conflicts with partners are expressed in many different ways as kidney pain. The kidneys, as a paired organ, represent personal contact and a relationship with a partner. This connection is demonstrated in simple everyday occurrences: sharing a drink is something that people often do when they meet each other. The extra liquid in the body then prompts the kidneys to act. The kidneys act because of our contact with other people. Problems with the kidneys mirror problems in our relationships with others.

A full bladder wants to be emptied; pressure waits to be relieved. Pressure always demands releases and relaxation. Pressure on the bladder can be felt acutely in certain situations, noticeably when we ourselves feel under pressure. Under the pretext of relieving oneself, it is possible to get rid of social pressure by leaving the room and transferring it to the other party.

Problems with the bladder are closely associated with problems in the exercise of power. Bed-wetting is often described as a kind of crying. It is frequently the reaction of a child put under constant pressure by its parents. The child has its 'revenge' by releasing the pressure in this way, and thus putting its parents under a different kind of pressure.

Where there are complications of the bladder, the patient should always try to find the source of the pressure that is making

Reflex zones of the urinary tract

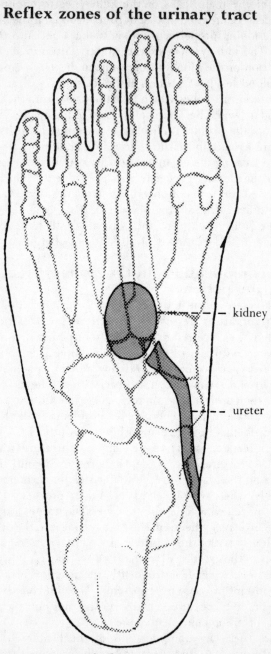

— — kidney

— — ureter

right foot—sole

Reflex zones of the urinary tract

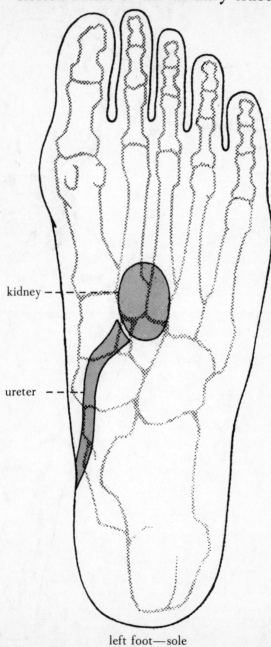

kidney

ureter

left foot—sole

Reflex zones of the urinary tract

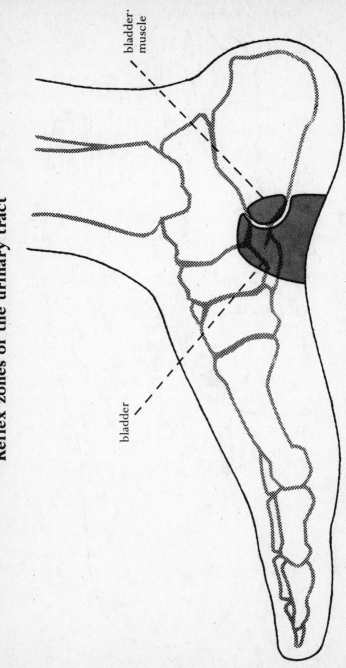

bladder muscle

bladder

inner aspect of the foot

him suffer. He should ask himself seriously what there is to cry about.

The zones of the lymphatic system

The lympathic system consists of numerous lymph glands, the spleen, thymus, tonsils and appendix.

The spleen is an important organ of self-defence, producing antibodies. It is a vascular organ, having a large arterial blood supply. It forms lymphocytes (white blood corpuscles) and breaks down old red blood corpuscles. But it is not a vital organ and if it has to be removed, its functions can be taken over by other organs (lymph nodes, liver and bone marrow).

Lymph is fluid drained from the body's tissue. It has a similar consistency to blood. Lymph flows through the body like a purifying stream. The lymphatic system plays a vital role in the body's defence and immunity system. Immunity is the ability of a body to use its own strength to keep it free of infection of pathogenic (disease-forming) micro-organisms, and from the influence of harmful foreign bodies and poisonous substances.

Referral zone	Position
upper lymphatics	in the webs of the toes (both sides of the feet)
tonsils	lateral aspect of both big toes at their base
axillary lymphatics	proximally to the zones of the shoulder joints
lymph nodes of the groin (inguinal lymphatics)	on the transverse stretch between the inner and outer ankle bones
lymphatics of the pelvis	at the heel, medially and laterally (see diagrams on page 112)
spleen	at the bases of 4th and 5th metatarsals on the sole of the left foot

The grip for decongesting the upper lymphatics is a gentle pull

Reflex zones of the lymphatic organs

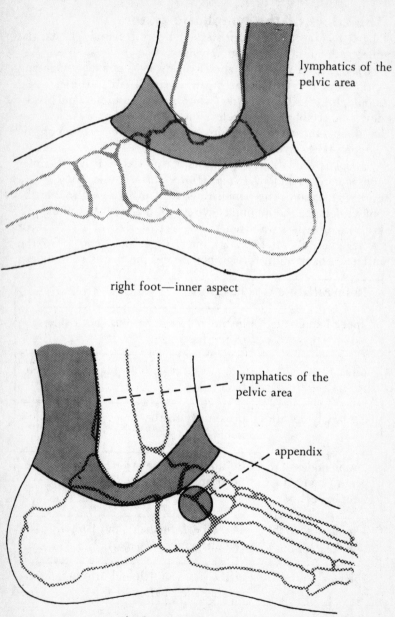

lymphatics of the
pelvic area

right foot—inner aspect

lymphatics of the
pelvic area

appendix

right foot—outer aspect

Reflex zones of the lymphatic organs

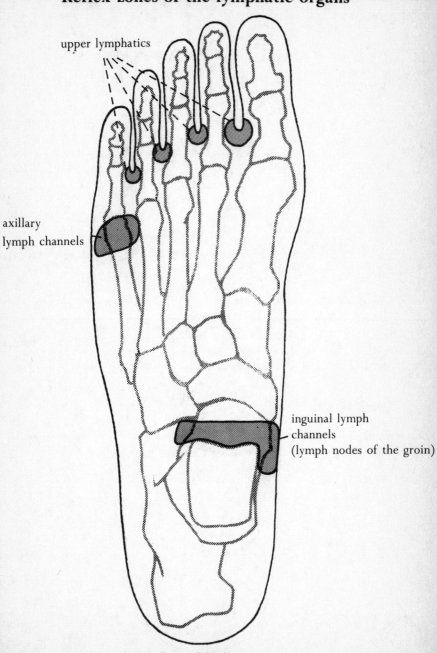

upper lymphatics

axillary
lymph channels

inguinal lymph
channels
(lymph nodes of the groin)

left foot—dorsal view

Reflex zones of the lymphatic organs

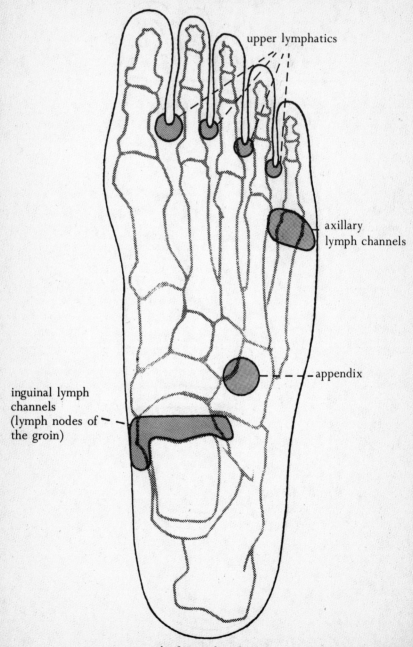

upper lymphatics

axillary
lymph channels

appendix

inguinal lymph
channels
(lymph nodes of
the groin)

right foot—dorsal view

Reflex zones of the lymphatic organs

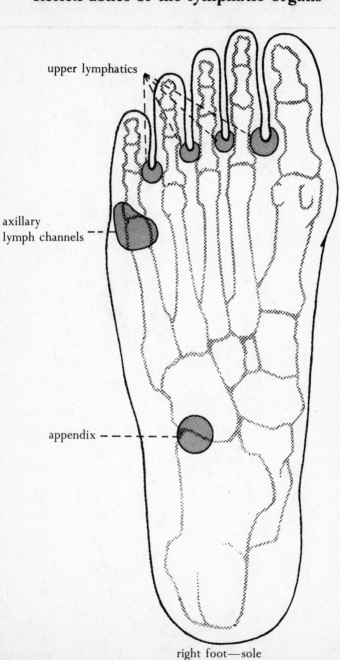

upper lymphatics

axillary
lymph channels ---

appendix - - - - -

right foot—sole

Reflex zones of the lymphatic organs

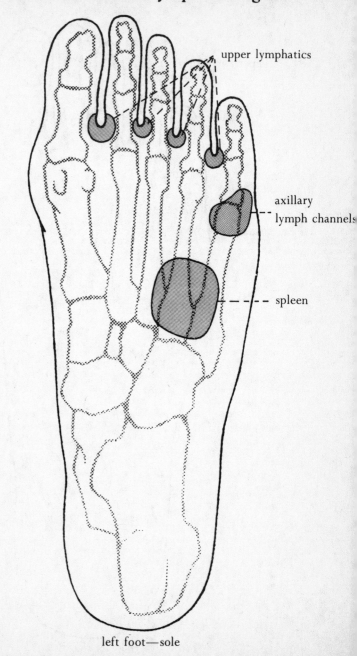

upper lymphatics

axillary
lymph channels

spleen

left foot—sole

with the thumb and forefinger on the webs, the folds of skin between the toes. They slip back into their original position when released.

In our practice we have found that large numbers of patients suffer from disturbances in the zones of the lymphatic system. This is due to the great demands put on the body's purifying system by bad diet, environmental pollution, the abuse of drugs and chemicals, and so on. Patients who have already had their tonsils removed often react just as strongly as those who have problems with their tonsils, when the appropriate zone is massaged. The reason for this is that the operation scar represents a disturbance in the energy field. The same disturbance is found with all scars on the body.

The reflex zone of the spleen is especially painful in the case of disorders of the upper abdomen and heart disease, allergies, abnormalities of the blood or lymph formation, and chronic and acute infections and inflammations.

The zones of the endocrine glands

Endocrine glands are those which secrete hormones directly into the blood system. They are the pituitary, thyroid, parathyroid, pancreas, adrenals, testes, ovaries, and many other small glands. The endocrine system covers the whole body and consists partly of ductless organs, partly of groups of hormone-producing cells in the organs (hypothalamus, epithelium of the intestine).

The hormones are complex chemical substances which, together with the nervous system, control the metabolic processes, growth and reproduction. They have no unifying structure or mechanism, but are rather blood-borne messengers. The hypothalamus plays an important role in controlling hormone secretion and the pituitary controls the other endocrine glands. The hormones affect the body processes, and also send reactions back to the glands that produced them, so they exert a two-way influence.

The body functions controlled by the hormones only run smoothly when the hormone supply is exactly regulated. Too much or too little will result in various illnesses characteristic of each malfunction.

If the thyroid is overactive (hyperthyroidism), the metabolic processes will be accelerated. Nutrients are burned up quickly and the subject shows nervous over-excitability. If the thyroid is underactive (hypothyroidism), there will be a reduction in the

Reflex zones of the endocrine glands

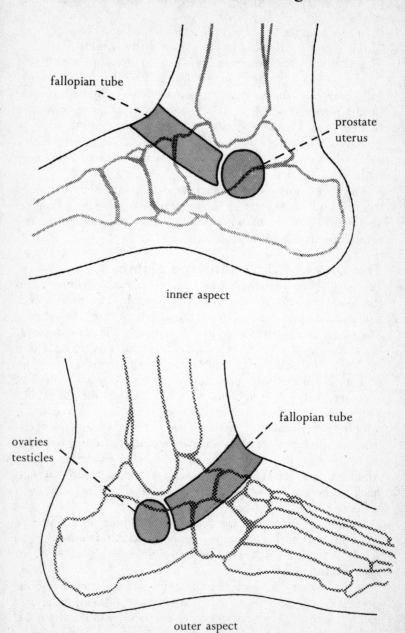

inner aspect

outer aspect

Reflex zones of the endocrine glands

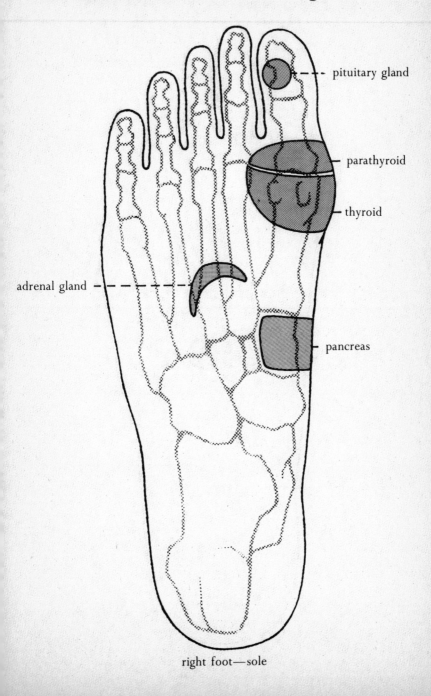

pituitary gland

parathyroid

thyroid

adrenal gland

pancreas

right foot—sole

Reflex zones of the endocrine glands

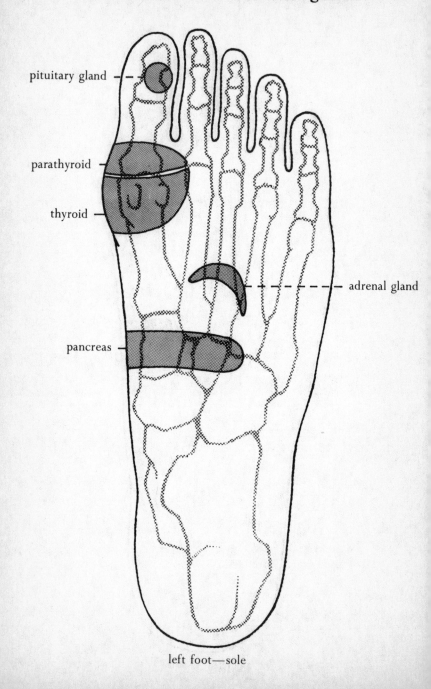

pituitary gland

parathyroid

thyroid

adrenal gland

pancreas

left foot—sole

metabolic rate. Nutrients are burned up more slowly, growth is retarded and there is general tiredness.

Referral zone	Position
pituitary	the ball of the big toe
thyroid	basal joint of the big toe (plantar and dorsal aspects)
pancreas	see under zones of the digestive system
adrenals	above Lisfranc's joint line on the soles of both feet in longitudinal zones 2 and 3 (see also under kidneys)
genital area uterus/vagina; prostate/testes	on both feet, across the 'ankle strap' (see diagrams on page 118)
ovaries	ankle bone, left and right feet

The zone of the pituitary can often be seen and felt as a small protrusion on the ball of the big toe. Care should be taken against over-stimulation in the treatment of the thyroid. Therapeutic stimulation to the reflex zones of the adrenals is very important in treating rheumatism and all kinds of allergies, because the adrenals produce the body's own supply of cortizone. Disorders of the gential area are extremely amenable to treatment by reflexology because of the holistic nature of the therapy.

Expectant mothers enjoying a trouble-free pregnancy can certainly benefit from reflex zone therapy, though this should be carried out with the knowledge and co-operation of the woman's doctor. For both mother and child, therapeutic stimuli that promote the body's functions and harmonize the life forces can do only good. Regular massages will have a relaxing effect and very often ensure an easy birth.

Women with premenstrual problems, such as extremely tender breasts and painful periods, can be relieved of these problems only after a few sessions of treatment.

In treating the zones of the endocrine system we are reminded very clearly of the necessity of orientating ourselves towards the root of the problem and its implications.

What disorders of the endocrine system reveal about the patient

People with over-active thyroid glands tend to be those who deny or suppress hostile feelings and a strong desire for independence. Sometimes they can be over-keen to help others, though they are actually incapable of helping even themselves. Many are very ambitious.

Much can be said about problems in the genital area. The aim of all-embracing sexuality is the unification of opposites. In our history and education, knowledge of the body and of sexuality has been considered reprehensible and even evil. It is an inherited attitude that causes many people a great deal of suffering. Dethlefsen and Dahlke write: 'What man can't do with his body, he will never manage with his head.' In other words, sexual problems have to be solved on the physical plane. Any attempts at resolving such conflicts mentally is doomed to failure.

If a woman has a problem with her periods, she is probably unhappy with her identity as a woman. Monthly periods are a rhythmical expression of fruitfulness and receptiveness. Every woman has to give herself to this cycle, and in doing so accepts her destiny as a woman. A woman who suffers because of her periods cannot accept her femininity; she feels devalued. Man and woman, masculine and feminine, giving and receiving: one is not better than the other, they are merely different.

The background to menstrual problems and many other sexual difficulties is an unresolved relationship to one's own sexuality. Having built up false ideas of the nature of femininity and masculinity, many people are afraid of giving themselves. Difficulties in sexual relations between men and women are mostly caused by fear. Sexuality fully experienced means that one loses control of oneself in orgasm. Many people are afraid of losing control, especially those who have been brought up on the principle of self-control. At the same time, losing control appears extremely attractive and desirable. Cramped and forced attempts are made to achieve the desired state, which by their very nature are blocks in the way of real letting go and opening up.

Determination and effort in the sexual realm are the beginning of a vicious circle. If the patient brings up his sexual problems, point him in the direction of the great mystery of letting go.

6

The Reflex Zones of the Hands

According to Dr Fitzgerald's concept of zone therapy, the hands also have reflex zones that correspond to different organs and parts of the body. Our experience shows better results in treating the feet than the hands, but work on the zones of the hands does have some advantages, particularly in self-treatment. In most cases, massaging the reflex zones of the hands makes a very good complement to foot massage.

The feet have always played a more important role than the hands in our concept of health. Cold feet and wet feet have been recognized from time immemorial to be potential causes of illness, and various treatments for the feet, such as mustard baths, have always been highly regarded. Going barefoot, walking in the dew and on gravel have been variously recommended at different times. Sebastian Kneipp in his book on hydrotherapy, *My Water Cure*, gives forty-six different treatments for the feet, but mentions the hands only once.

We advocate working on the reflex zones of the hands primarily for self-treatment. Treatment is similar to that of the feet. We begin with the spine, then work through the zones of the head, respiratory system, heart and liver, and on to the digestive tract and the zones of the lymphatic organs. Especially useful for self-treatment are the zones of the spine and the solar plexus. Massaging these can relieve nervousness. A passifying grip on the zones of the bronchials can be very effective in treating an attack of coughing. Blood pressure can be regulated with the pincer grip—a gentle massage with thumb and forefinger, pulling the flesh on the metacarpals all the way along the hand to the fingers, and releasing it so that it springs back. This grip should be repeated 15–20 times on each hand, several times a day. This massage brings about a general harmonization, whether the problem is one of high or low blood pressure.

Reflex zones of the hand

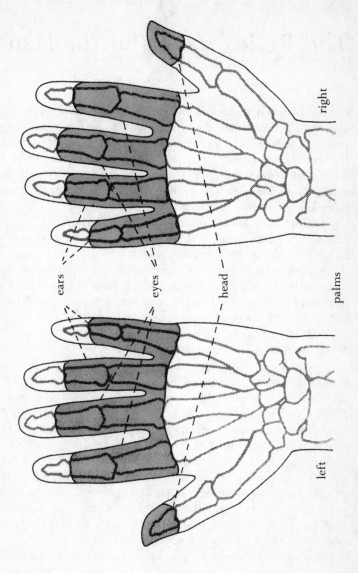

ears

eyes

head

right

palms

left

Reflex zones of the hand

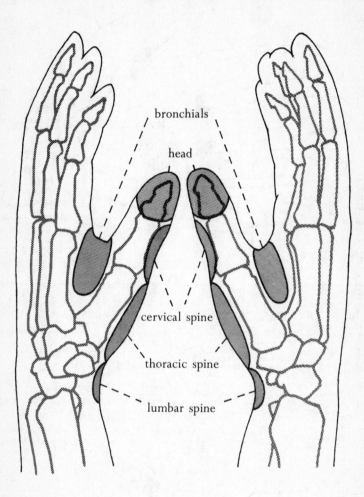

left hand   right hand

Reflex zones of the hand

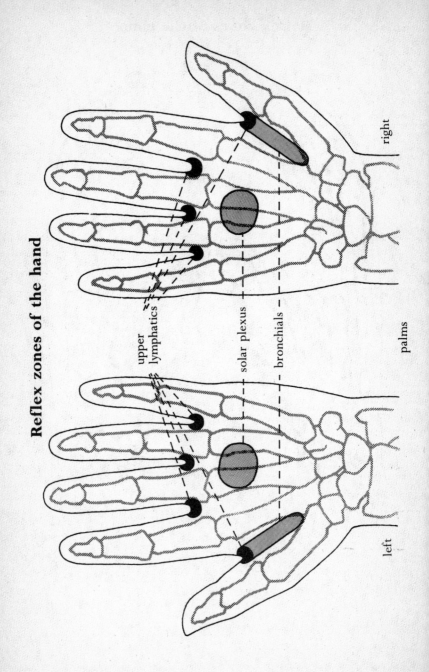

upper
lymphatics

solar plexus

bronchials

right

left

palms

Reflex zones of the hand

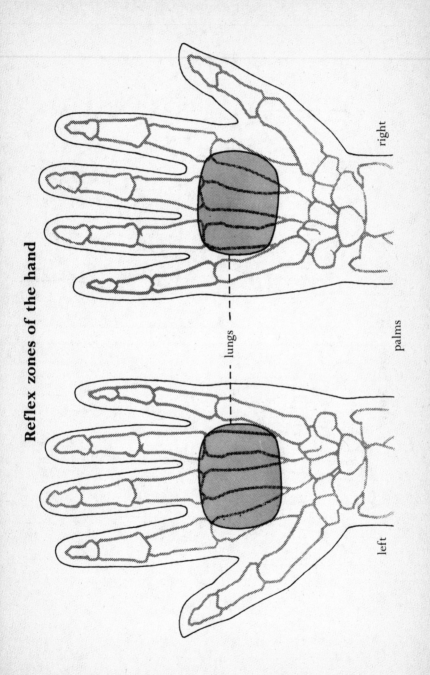

right

palms

lungs

left

Reflex zones of the hand

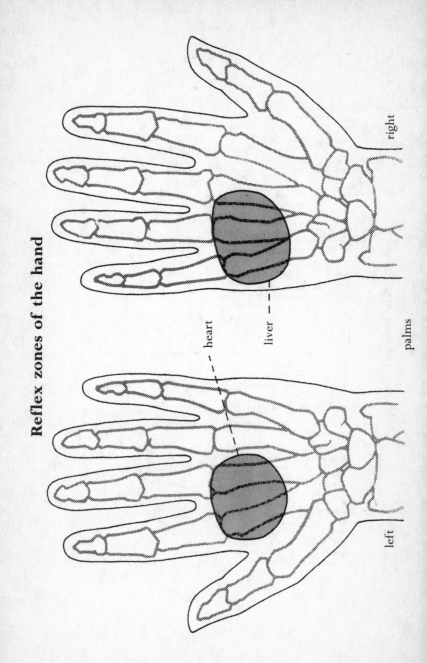

heart

liver

right

palms

left

Reflex zones of the hand

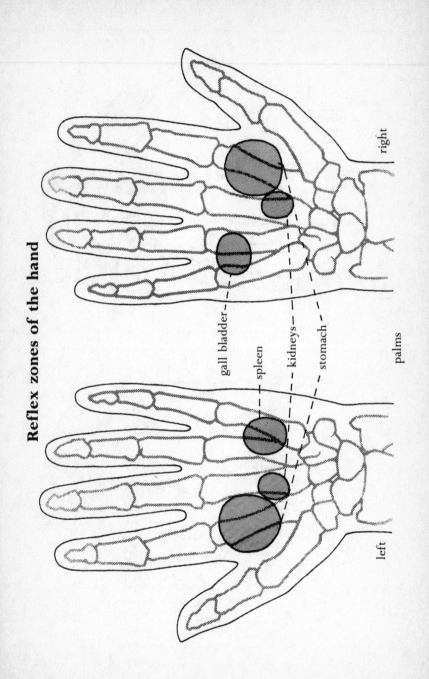

gall bladder

spleen

kidneys

stomach

right

palms

left

Reflex zones of the hand

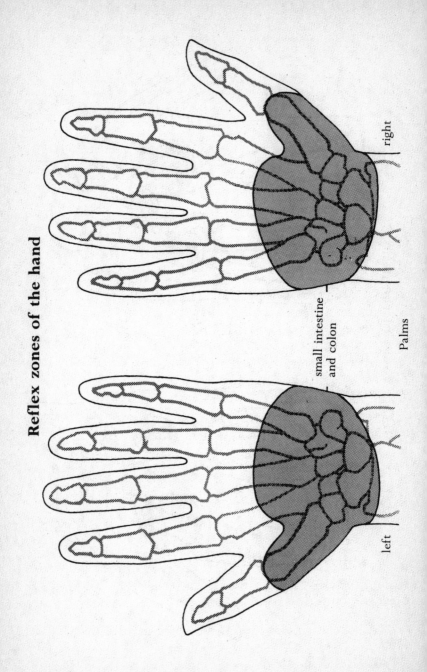

small intestine
and colon

right

left

Palms

7

Reflexology: A Course of Treatment

Reflexology is primarily a treatment that promotes and maintains health. Anyone who practises it is a guardian of health before he is a healer. We have all become accustomed to looking after our cars and taking them for regular services. We take far less care of our own bodies than we do of many of the machines that we use from day to day, yet our bodies have got to last all over lives.

Reflexology offers an excellent opportunity to take some preventative measures. Minor disturbances can quickly be sorted out and the constant harmonizing of the body's energies has a tangible positive effect on spiritual and physical well-being and results in a more lively attitude to life. It is very important to remain active, to keep going and maintain a balance at the same time. It is rather like riding a bicycle—if you stop, you fall off. We have developed a false idea of security—we associate safety mainly with being at rest. Yet there is no rest in life. Where there is rest, there is no movement, and where there is no movement, there is no life. We must fight daily to maintain our balance and we must let our life forces fight for us. Massaging the reflex zones can improve our awareness of our own life forces and influence them in a positive way.

In this section we outline a general course of treatment, detailing the most important steps along the way and drawing attention to possible causes and reactions where appropriate. Obviously it is impossible to cover every eventuality because of the very individual nature of the treatment. Each person must be seen as a new encounter with unique life forces. The basic principle underlying the notes that follow is the one introduced at the beginning of this book and followed through the discussion of the reflex zones.

Despite the schematic divisions in this chapter, the treatment is not symptom-orientated. We do not concentrate immediately on the disturbed zone. First we must relax the patient and restore harmony by massaging the zones of the spine. This calms the nervous system and allows the patient to open himself up and speak about the underlying causes of his problems.

In each encounter with a patient, and each time we give reflex zone massage, we must renew our awareness of responsibility to the patient. Trust in the methods and principles of therapy is more important for the patient than keeping an eye on any ultimate goals of treatment. We must keep constantly in mind the fact that human problems cannot be solved by technical means, they can be solved only in human terms. We have forgotten to a large extent how to talk to one another and how to understand each other. The sick person speaks to us in his own language and we must learn to understand what he says. The patient, in turn, must learn a new attitude to self-expression, and a new relationship to himself. Our understanding can only grow gradually, with each human encounter. We can learn most of all from our dealings with other people. We must always be ready to learn.

General sequence of zones to be treated

1. The spine.
2. The head, sinuses, teeth, eyes, and ears.
3. The upper lymphatics.
4. The breathing, nose, throat, tonsils, bronchials, and lungs.
5. The heart.
6. The diaphragm.
7. The digestion: mouth, teeth, oesophageal sphincter (entrance to stomach), stomach, pyloric sphincter (exit from stomach), spleen, liver, gall bladder, small intestine, colon, pancreas, intestines (general), appendix, rectum, and anus.
8. The kidneys and adrenals.
9. The bladder and prostate.
10. The ovaries and womb.
11. The endocrine glands.
12. The lymphatic organs.
13. The joints.
14. The musculature.
15. Solar plexus relaxation grip.

Zone	Indication
The spine	Begin by massaging the spine from the coccyx upwards. With a supple, gentle, and at the same time dynamic grip, massage the spine again, this time from the cervical spine down

to the coccyx. Repeat this massaging, 3–5 times changing direction each time. When massaging the spine, the therapist will be able to detect the first signs of any disturbances, because the central nervous system serves all the important organs. The downwards massage stimulates the nerves leaving the spine and has a relaxing and harmonizing effect. A large number of disorders are caused by nervous blockages due to static build-ups in the spine, and can be relieved by reflex zone massage.

The head and sinuses	The skull is massaged with the sinuses, then the brain and the neck. When you get to the neck, move the massaging thumb slightly from side to side in a rocking motion. It is important to get the dosage of massage to the pituitary right. It needs to be functioning perfectly to be able to regulate the hormones in the body. Children are especially receptive to a gentle and sensitive massage of the pituitary reflex zones. Women with certain forms of infertility also respond well to massage of this area because the pituitary regulates the sex hormones. Some kinds of flu benefit from a massage of the zones of the nose and throat. Special attention should of course be paid to the zones of the head when the patient complains of any kind of head pain, though the causes of migraine need to be searched for elsewhere, as already described. Special care must be taken with the zones of the nervous system.
The teeth	Bad teeth are known to be the malicious root of many an illness. If a tooth shows an overreaction to a change in temperature (hot or cold drinks), it can be treated with a passifying massage grip. But if the therapist discovers a bad tooth, with infection or pus, dental treatment will be necessary. To try to relieve the pain in this case would be to treat the symptom and not the cause of the problem. If a

The autonomic nervous system

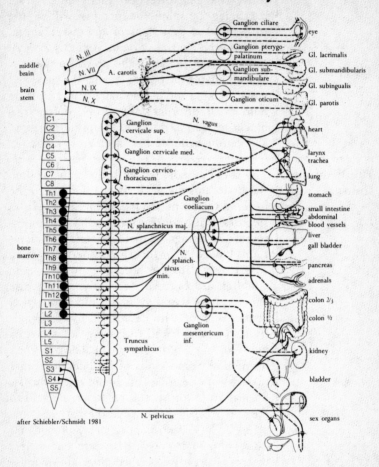

after Schiebler/Schmidt 1981

►— parasympathetic nerves (responsible for energy saving, relaxation, recovery and recuperation)

●— sympathetic nerves (responsible for spending energy, activity, tension)

Because the organs are so richly supplied with nerves, massaging the reflex zones of the spine is often as effective as massaging the zones corresponding to the organs. Treating the central nervous system in the spine by massaging the zones on the feet brings about optimum harmonisation.

	zone reacts painfully, though the corresponding tooth has already been removed, then it is the scar left behind that is acting as a disturbance in the energy field, and this can be treated.
The eyes	The reflex zones of the eyes in the 2nd and 3rd longitudinal zones have shown themselves very amenable to treatment after operations and in the improvement of short-sightedness (zone 2) and long-sightedness (zone 3). By stimulating these zones the musculature of the eyes can be strengthened, which can also result in improved sight.
The ears	The inner ear (longitudinal zone 4) can be successfully treated for buzzing in the ears, disturbed balance and a certain type of deafness.
The upper lymphatics	After massaging the zones of the head, it is important to go on to the upper lymphatics. A massage to this zone will ensure the free flow of toxins from the area. If this is not done, a blockage of lymph could lead to new problems and cause headaches. In cases of asthma, hayfever and other allergies, the webs between the 2nd and 3rd or 3rd and 4th toes will be particularly sensitive. Adequate application of the pincer grip to activate the lympathics is then especially important.
The breathing, nose and throat	The zones of the respiratory system are treated on the dorsal side of the foot. The plantar aspect of this area has too high a concentration of the nervous system.
The tonsils	The vocal cords can also be treated in a massage of the zones of the tonsils. Good results are often obtained with hoarseness.
The bronchials	The bronchials are treated on the dorsal side of

	the feet with a massage in a proximal direction.
The lungs	The zones of the lungs can be massaged on both dorsal and plantar sides of the feet.
The heart	If disturbances are found in the reflex zones of the heart, the patient must be examined by a doctor. If the therapist is working with a doctor he can positively influence the regeneration of the heart musculature in a heart-attack patient and help restore the heart to normal functioning. Disturbances in the zones of the heart can point to upsets in the patient's emotional life. They can also be caused by breathing problems (tension between the ribs). In treating the zones of the heart, the therapist must bear in mind the holistic nature of reflexology—a pain in the heart can mean exactly that: that the patient is 'sick at heart'.
The diaphragm	A constricted diaphragm need not necessarily imply problems with the respiratory systems. It can equally well point to a disorder of the stomach or the intestines (wind). It can be treated by releasing the tension between the ribs. Disturbances in the zone of the diaphragm can also be aided by stimulating the zone of the solar plexus. It is interesting to note that children who develop asthma often complain of stomach ache first and that treatment of the zone of the appendix has been effective in these cases.
The digestion: mouth, teeth, and oesophagus	Treat the same zones as for the bronchials.
The oesophageal sphincter (entrance to the stomach)	On the left foot. If the cardia is slightly inflamed, the passifying grip should be applied.

The stomach	Acute gastric attacks need to be countered with a stationary grip exerting a passifying influence; digestive problems due to lack of acid in the stomach need stimulation. Too much acid is also treated by stimulation, which in this case encourages the stomach to regulate its acid production itself. Special care is needed in the treatment of ulcers—massage can cause them to rupture. A 'nervous' stomach needs a stationary passifying grip.
The pyloric sphincter (exit from the stomach)	On the right foot. Disturbances in the zone of the cardia and pylorus are usually due to inflammation.
The spleen	On the left foot. The spleen plays an important role in the body's defence mechanism (immune system). This reflex zone should normally be activated gently.
The liver	If a patient is suffering from hepatitis, the condition of the liver can be quite dramatically improved by massaging its reflex zone. The function of the liver as an excretory organ is important for the metabolism and for the circulation. Stimulation of the liver can be very beneficial in treating tiredness and depression. Use a pincer grip with thumb and forefinger and draw the flesh firmly but gently along the metatarsals on the dorsal side of the feet in a distal direction to stimulate the circulation.
The gall bladder	Needs to be treated with care. Massage can trigger wandering gall stones. If in doubt, always consult a doctor before continuing treatment. The stimulation of the zone of the gall bladder is important in relieving indigestion. Use a pincer grip of thumb and forefinger to stimulate both plantar and dorsal sides of the feet. When treating the gall bladder, it will

	be noticed that its position can vary quite considerably from one person to the next (3rd, 4th or 5th longitudinal zone).
The small intestine	The zones of the small intestine are surrounded by the separate sections of the zones of the colon.
The colon	The colon is massaged following its shape: ascending colon, transverse colon and descending colon, leading to the anus.
The pancreas	Massaged together with the stomach. The pancreas needs to be treated with special care in diabetic patients, as insulin shock can easily be triggered off. In this case the patient should be given sugar, or grape sugar.
The intestines (general)	Need activating to counteract problems with the digestion. Should be activated to treat diarrhoea and constipation. Intestinal problems need to be investigated in conjunction with the patient's diet and lifestyle.
The appendix	An inflamed appendix should be treated with a passifying grip. The zone of the appendix offers an excellent opportunity for diagnosis. If the patient has a pain you suspect to be in the appendix, and which disappears for a short period when you stimulate the zone of the appendix, you can be sure that the appendix is inflamed.
The rectum	The reflex zones of the rectum are to be found, once again symmetrically, on the left and right foot.
The anus	Disturbances in the reflex zone of the sphincter point to haemorrhoids, cramps or eczema. A passifying grip on the reflex zone often results in a warm feeling in the anus and a relaxation of pressure. Do not forget to treat

	the pelvic lymph glands in this context.
The kidneys	The same word of warning applies here as with the gall bladder—kidney stones can be set wandering by the massage of these zones. Massage in the zones of the urinary tract should move both distally and proximally because the kidneys expel waste and the bladder draws it up. The therapist must be conscious of the limitations of this treatment: a loosened stone can cause a blockage and cut off a kidney completely. If kidney stones are suspected, consult a doctor. The true master of the therapy will always recognize his limitations.
The adrenals	The stimulation of the adrenals is important with allergies because they are responsible for producing the body's natural supply of pain-killing cortizone. Stimulation of the adrenal glands can also greatly improve low blood pressure.
The bladder	Bladder function can be stimulated, but the sphincter needs a passifying stationary grip, especially in cases of bed-wetting. Bed-wetting is determined by other factors, both psychological and social. In children, the relationship between the child and its parents should be investigated.
The prostate	Many urinary problems can be improved with sensitive massage that stimulates the circulation.
The ovaries/ uterus	Irregular periods and period pains can both benefit from reflexology. Normal rhythm can be restored and pain relieved. In the treatment of irregular periods, the pituitary should also be treated because of its role in hormone production and regulation. Here, as with many other disorders, psychological and social

factors should be taken into consideration.

The endocrine glands	The reflex zones of the endocrine glands are stimulated according to their function, and how much attention this requires. Because the workings of these glands are very complex, quite a while may elapse between treatment and reaction. Allergies may be successfully treated by massage. Gentle stimulation to the thyroid can also normalize the functioning of this gland.
The lymphatic organs	When decongesting the lymphatic organs with the pincer grip, care should be taken to start with the upper lymphatics. The reflex zones of the pelvis and the lymphatic organs situated there are mostly treated last. If necessary, the lymphatics can be treated several times in one session, but in any case massage of the zones of the lymphatics should always end the session to ensure the elimination of harmful substances from the body. The grip for decongesting the upper lymphatics has already been described in some detail: it involves pulling on the webs between the toes. Decongestion of the lympathics of the pelvis is achieved with a gentle pincer grip pulling rhythmically along the Achilles tendon towards the heel. It can be done with the thumb and forefinger, or by using both hands.
The joints	Joints and musculature will of course be treated all through the massage. If massage indicates problems with a joint in one of the reflex zones, the patient will probably feel a sharp stabbing pain, which will enable you to pinpoint the exact location of the trouble. Hold a steady passifying grip on the trouble spot for a while—in most cases the patient will feel immediate increased mobility in the joint referred to, except if the ligament has been torn or a similar injury sustained. In

treating tennis elbow (*epicondylitis humeri*), make sure to include the cervical spine, chest, shoulder and upper arm in the treatment, as well as the elbow itself. Tennis elbow can also be successfully treated with acupuncture.

The musculature	Muscle tonus can be greatly improved by stimulation through reflex zone therapy. As the musculature supports the skeletal framework of the body, treatment of the muscles must be included as appropriate in any treatment of the bones (for example, backache in the small of the back will call for treatment of the musculature of the stomach as well as of the spine). If there is a general muscle tension it is always an indication of the patient's psychological state, which will need to be investigated. Tension in the neck and shoulders signifies that the patient is weighed down with problems.

Though each illness may seem to be a phenomenon that is specific and infinitely repeatable—the same in all afflicted patients—it is important not to rob the patient of his individuality. The responsible therapist will never reduce his relationship with the patient to one of predictable biophysical/chemical stimulus and reaction. The laws of physics and chemistry only come completely into their own when the body has no life left in it. The corpse will uphold all the laws of science. As long as the body has the power of life in it, a different set of laws applies—laws about which we know far too little.

No one should believe that it is possible to become a specialist just by reading a book. Reflexology is a method of healing based on thousands of years of experience and can be learned only by practice. To ignore its limitations is irresponsible and can be dangerous. Learning by experience is a slow process, but it is ultimately rewarding, and anyone who wants to practise re-flexology will have to go through it.

There have been moves towards privatization and monopoly of reflexology. Such moves will always be doomed to fail because the principles of reflexology are deeply rooted in a desire for the common good. Anyone who holds by this will want as many people as possible to learn about the various methods of healing and to put them into practice. Reflexology is a method of promoting good health and preventing ill health and, as such, is not the province of the specialist alone—it is simple enough to be learned and applied by anyone. The main thing is to understand the principles on which reflexology is based and to put this understanding into practice. That is why this book has been written.

8

Some Case Histories

It took a long time to decide whether or not to include examples of case histories from our practice in this book. Some books give detailed and very dramatic accounts of how patients have been cured, and there is often a suggestion of self-congratulation here, which we wished to avoid. Much more dangerous, however, is the notion that such case histories might serve as 'recipes' to be followed in treating similar cases.

Eventually we decided to give a few brief but striking examples, because we believe that the reader has a right to know the vast potential of a therapy that works with the body's own life forces.

A 64-year-old woman had been suffering with asthma for thirty-five years, with occasional very severe attacks. After twenty treatments the asthma disappeared—she has had no sign of it now for four years.

A 13-year-old child had been suffering asthma attacks for five years. His body had grown intolerant of drugs and he could not take cortizone. After ten treatments a scar in the pelvic region was located and the disturbance in the energy field defused. The child has not suffered from asthma since.

If shingles is caught right at the beginning it can mostly be cured after between three and five treatments.

A 70-year-old patient was told by her doctor that she had ruptured her groin on both sides. After fifteen treatments she felt a great deal better and after ten further treatments, during which she felt a strong pulling and a warmth in her groin, the hernias were healed.

A patient who had sustained head injuries from an explosion during the war had had an operation in which a silver plate was inserted. He could not speak or walk beyond about five or ten steps. Visual and tactile examination of his feet showed a massive disturbance in the pituitary, cranium and brain. There were also disorders in the cervical, thoracic and lumbar regions of the spine. After five treatments he could already utter a few sentences. This success freed other energy blocks in his body. He had a great determination to recover, and after a further twelve treatments he was able to walk several kilometres.

A 67-year-old patient had suffered a heart attack after a holiday in the mountains. Six months after a stay in hospital, he came to visit us. He had still not fully recovered. We gave his whole body a very thorough treatment and after about twenty sessions no trace of the heart attack showed up on the EEG. The patient had made a complete recovery.

A 9-year-old child had great difficulty in concentrating at school and could therefore not do the work required of him. A visual examination showed disturbances in the spine, pituitary and upper lymphatics. After a few sessions the disorders decreased and the child already showed less fear of school. After nine sessions, the child was able to do his homework and school exercises unaided. He developed very good powers of concentration and had no more problems at school.

A baby of 3 months had not been able to pass motions unaided. A visual examination showed a swelling in the zone of the intestines. During the very first treatment, the baby passed a motion himself and after three further sessions the workings of his intestines had become completely regular.

A cyclist taking part in an international racing tour complained of a sharp pain in the knee after completing a gruelling uphill section of the circuit. After a short while, his knee was badly swollen. A visual and tactile examination of the zone of the knee showed no disturbances whatsoever. But a major disturbance was found in the zone of one of his teeth. It was recommended that he have the tooth out right away. The following day the cyclist had a badly swollen cheek, but his knee had completely recovered and he was able to continue the race.

A 30-year-old woman came to see us, complaining of a constant cold. No treatment that she had tried so far had been of the slightest use. The only disturbed zones were those of the ovaries, oviducts and womb. She had been fitted with a contraceptive coil and her body was clearly reacting against it. The patient was recommended to have the coil removed. Three further treatments were sufficient to restore harmony and the cold cleared up completely.

A 27-year-old patient suffered from bad attacks of migraine, some of which lasted for up to four days. A tactile examination showed disturbances in the zones of the cervical and lumbar spines, pelvis and intestines. After seven treatments, the patient remained free of attacks for six months. After three further series of five treatments, the migraines cleared up completely.

A 40-year-old patient had bruises all over his body after a car accident. His rib-cage and abdomen were particularly painful and had not responded to medication. A tactile examination showed massive disturbances between the ribs and in the musculature of the stomach. After two long sessions of very thorough treatment, the patient was completely free of pain.

A 23-year-old quadraplegic patient had violent headaches on one side of the head and suffered from constipation and profuse sweating. Because she was quadraplegic it was difficult to reach any conclusions after a tactile examination, but after seven general harmonizing treatments her headaches disappeared, the bowels became regular and the excessive sweating stopped.

Potted histories such as these could fill a book in themselves. Every reader will doubtless know of other cases that sound incredible at first, but are in fact testimonies to the mysterious nature of the power of life.

9

Questions and Answers About Reflex Zone Massage

Q What is reflex zone massage?
A It is a form of treatment whereby zones on the feet are massaged to stimulate the flow of life forces in the body and improve the functioning of the organism.

Q How does the treatment work?
A There is still no complete explanation for the success of reflexology. There have been many attempts at explanation and they are all correct in their way, but no mechanical analogy, such as crystalline deposits or blocks in the nervous system, can really give any idea of the scope the therapy offers. What we can say is that an image of the body is projected onto the feet, and that by massaging the feet we are treating the patient as a whole being.

Q Who administers the treatment?
A Reflexology is basically an inherited folk medicine and has been used from time immemorial by people who want to look after their own health. The potential of reflexology as a healing art has been developed in recent times and there are now expert reflexologists who have been trained to treat the body by foot massage. The trained therapist will always work in collaboration with a doctor if he suspects or discovers a particular complaint. As a method of preserving the health and preventing disease, the practice of reflexology is open to any responsible person who cares to learn about it.

Q What makes a patient suited to treatment by reflexology?
A It is primarily healthy people who are massaged. Reflexology is first and foremost a method of maintaining health and preventing illness. But if disturbances are found in the zones massaged, the reflexologist is well placed to provide the therapeutic stimulus necessary to mobilize the body's own powers of healing.

Q How does the reflexologist work?
A The therapist uses his hands, and only his hands, to trigger the therapeutic stimuli. In particular, he uses a dynamic and sensitive movement of the thumb.

Q What exactly does the therapist treat?
A In the narrow sense of the word, the therapist treats only the feet of the patient. But reflexology is always concerned with the whole person as a unity of body and soul and recognizes that physical problems can have many different causes. So it does not treat illness in isolation, but concentrates on the patient's whole person and personality. It is not concerned with symptoms, but treats the trouble at its root. In other words, it is a holistically orientated therapy, like, for example, homoeopathy.

Q What can be deduced from pain in certain zones on the feet?
A If the patient feels pain when the therapist is massaging a certain zone, it means that there is a disturbance, or a build-up of pressure or blockage in the corresponding referral zone in the body. No exact conclusions about the nature of the disturbance can be drawn. We can, however, detect disturbances that will not be evident in laboratory testing. In such cases we can help the body to help itself before the disturbance manifests itself as an illness.

Q Can anyone be treated by reflexology?
A There are some cases in which it is not advisable to treat a patient with reflexology. Details of these are given in the book. In general, however, no one is excluded by age, sex, or by the nature of their complaint.

Q How long does the treatment last?
A The first session lasts for about 45 minutes, and the following massage sessions for about 30 minutes each. A treatment generally comprises 8–12 sessions, according to the patient's reactions and progress. We usually recommend that healthy people should have two courses of treatment a year to recharge and stabilize the energy flow through their bodies. Apart from this, anyone can have reflex zone therapy whenever he feels like it, or feels he needs it.

Q How does the patient react to having the reflex zones on his feet massaged?

A   The reactions vary as much as the individuals treated. The therapist will be able to tell if he is exceeding a desirable dose of treatment. One of the things he has to learn is how to interpret the patient's reactions during treatment and to adapt the massage accordingly. Not knowing what the patient's reactions mean can lead to problems. It is therefore the first commandment to work gently and sensitively on the person's feet to avoid unexpected reactions. On no account should the therapist have his determination set on forcing the person to get better! This only causes tension on both sides and hinders the free flow of energy The more sensitive the massage, the more effective it will ultimately prove. One common general reaction is a feeling of warmth, relaxation and improved circulation in the corresponding zone of the body.

Q   Is it possible to treat yourself with reflexology?
A   Self-treatment does have disadvantages which make it a less efficient form of therapy than treating someone else. One very important factor is missing in self-treatment is relaxation. It is easy to misinterpret your own reactions, and in self-treatment there is no exchange of energy with the therapist. This exchange of energy is fundamental to the success of the treatment. Therefore if possible, it is much better to entrust yourself to someone who will massage your feet with care, and with whom you can relax. If partners practice reflexology on each other, or within the family group or circle of friends, the intelligent physical contact can strengthen bonds of trust between them.

Q   There is a range of gadgets and mechanical aids available today that claim to be effective in reflex zone massage. How useful are they?
A   Responsible therapists recommend patients to steer clear of such gadgets, and would never use them themselves. If mechanical aids are used, it is impossible to gauge the patient's reactions. The hand of the experienced therapist can be very deft in its stimulation and very sensitive in registering the patient's response. No mechanical implement could replace it. Gadgets such as foot rollers may, if used in moderation, stimulate the circulation, but a healthier and better way of doing this is to walk barefoot on the grass, an activity that stimulates the soles of the feet in the most natural possible way.

Q How does one recognize a good therapist?
A In her book *Reflexology: A Patient's Guide* (Thorsons) Nicola Hall says: 'Once the decision to try reflexology treatment has been taken, then the next important step is to try to find a good practitioner of the method. The recent growing interest in the alternative therapies has led to an increase in the number of people practising the various therapies and also an increase in the number of training courses available for them. This has its advantages and disadvantages and with reflexology there is much variation in the qualifications and proficiency of practitioners. In addition, in Britain at present there are no laws governing the practice of the alternative therapies, so there is nothing to stop an unqualified person setting up a practice for any of them, provided that they do not call themselves a doctor of medicine without having the appropriate medical qualification.

Often reflexology is one treatment offered by an alternative therapist along with other therapies and this can sometimes be useful. It is important in these instances, though, that if reflexology treatment is offered that it is given in its full form with massage of all the areas of the feet and not just massage of a few areas. Some therapists may use reflexology as a means of diagnosis and then treat with other methods.

There are several training schools for reflexology, some of which teach to a higher standard than others. The first reflexology training school established in Britain was started by the late Doreen E. Bayly who having run training courses since the early 1960s both in Britain and on the continent formed her own school in 1968 called the Bayly School of Reflexology. The School still runs regular training courses and students have to pass a written and practical test before being issued with a Certificate. The format for the courses has changed over the years and the tests for a Certificate were first introduced in 1980. A few other training schools make their students pass tests before issuing a Certificate, but some training schools just offer a Certificate of Attendance. It does, however, seem vital that students receive a sound training if they are to see patients on a professional basis.

The main training schools are able to give the names and addresses of trained practitioners in the various areas of the country and there is now a considerable number of people practising reflexology. Practitioners are allowed to advertise and names and addresses may be found in health magazines and sometimes in local newspapers. A local health shop will also probably be aware of the practitioners in their area. An advertisement does not necessarily mean that the person advertising is qualified, so it is most important that when contacting someone with a view to receiving treatment that they are asked where they trained and perhaps the length of their training—anyone properly qualified will not feel embarrassed to give this information. The other initial question must be about the cost involved for treatment, remembering that a course of treatment will probably be necessary. If an appointment is made, it is wise to look at the practitioner's Certificate at the first visit to make sure that they are genuine.

No elaborate equipment is required to give reflexology so it is not uncommon to find practitioners working from a room in their own home. A comfortable recliner-type chair should be used for the treatment and if this type of facility is not available then the treatment is not being approached in a very professional way. Many centres for alternative therapies have now been established around the country and it is usual for a reflexology practitioner to be included among the therapists working at such centres.'

The important thing is that you should be with a person and in a place that make you feel relaxed and comfortable. Neither of you should be pressed for time. The most essential thing is that you are both aware that this is a holistic treatment and that it calls for a responsible and caring attitude on the part of the one giving the massage. Reflexology cannot be reduced to the mastery of a technique. If you decide to be treated by a specialist, make it clear that you already know something about reflexology. A good therapist will always be frank and will appreciate frankness from you too. It is as well to remember that any therapist, however good he may be, will make no progress unless the patient is co-operative. Long-term success will come only if therapist and patient are both attuned to the treatment.

The Reflex Zones of the Feet

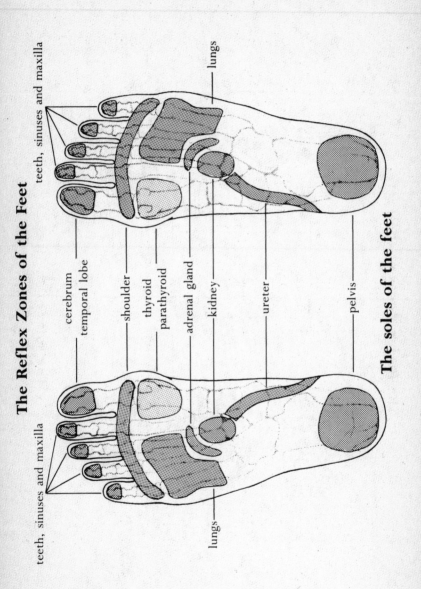

teeth, sinuses and maxilla

teeth, sinuses and maxilla

lungs

cerebrum
temporal lobe

shoulder

thyroid
parathyroid

adrenal gland

kidney

ureter

pelvis

lungs

The soles of the feet

The Reflex Zones of the Feet

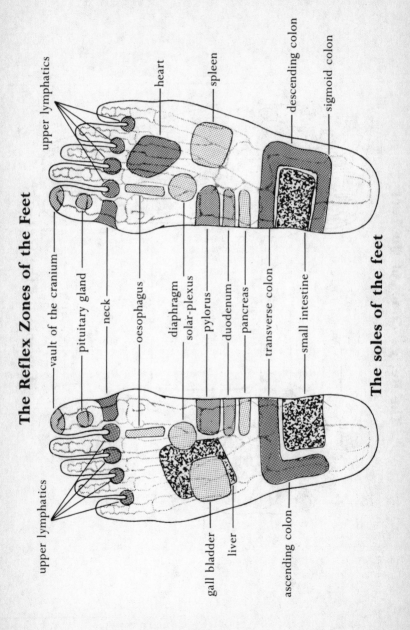

The soles of the feet

upper lymphatics

vault of the cranium
pituitary gland
neck
oesophagus
diaphragm
solar-plexus
pylorus
duodenum
pancreas
transverse colon
small intestine

heart
spleen
descending colon
sigmoid colon

upper lymphatics

gall bladder
liver
ascending colon

The Reflex Zones of the Feet

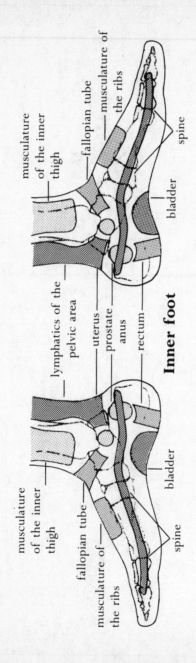

musculature of the inner thigh

musculature of the ribs

fallopian tube

spine

bladder

lymphatics of the pelvic area

uterus

prostate

anus

rectum

musculature of the inner thigh

fallopian tube

musculature of the ribs

spine

bladder

Inner foot

The Reflex Zones of the Feet

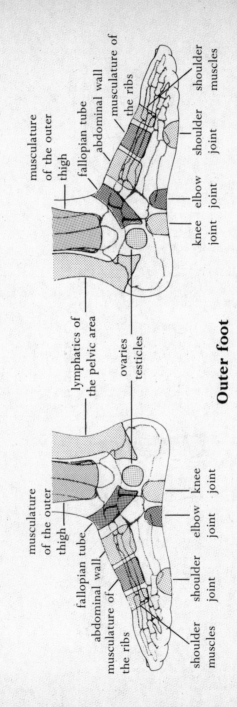

musculature
of the outer
thigh

fallopian tube
abdominal wall
musculature of
the ribs

shoulder
muscles

shoulder
joint

elbow
joint

knee
joint

lymphatics of
the pelvic area

ovaries
testicles

musculature
of the outer
thigh

fallopian tube
abdominal wall
musculature of
the ribs

shoulder
muscles

shoulder
joint

elbow
joint

knee
joint

Outer foot

The Reflex Zones of the Feet

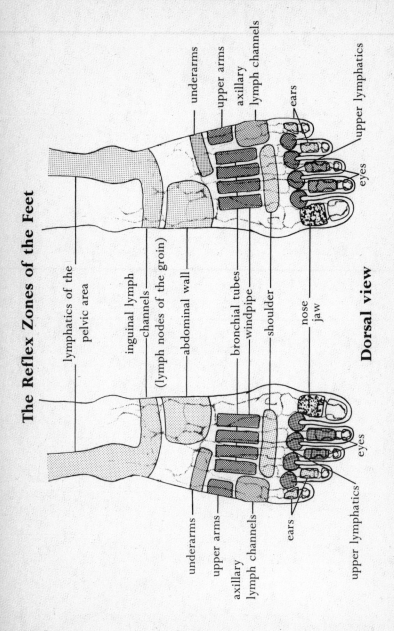

lymphatics of the
pelvic area

inguinal lymph
channels
(lymph nodes of the groin)

abdominal wall

bronchial tubes

windpipe

shoulder

nose
jaw

underarms

upper arms

axillary
lymph channels

ears

upper lymphatics

eyes

underarms

upper arms

axillary
lymph channels

ears

upper lymphatics

eyes

Dorsal view

Bibliography

Bertherat, Therese: *Der entspannte Körper,* Munich 1982.

Carter, Mildred: *Helping Yourself with Foot Reflexology,* Prentice–Hall 1960.

Dethlefsen, Thorwald and Dahlke, Rüdiger: *Krankheit als Weg,* Munich 1983.

Faller, Adolf: *Der Körper des Menschen,* Stuttgart 1976.

Fitzgerald, William H. and Bowers, Edwin F.: *Zone Therapy,* California 1917.

Hess, Werner: *Homöopathische Hausapotheke,* Stuttgart 1981.

Ingham, Eunice D.: *Stories the Feet Can Tell,* Rochester 1938.

Ingham, Eunice D.: *Stories the Feet Have Told,* Rochester 1983.

Jaffe, Dennis T.: *Kräfte der Selbstheilung,* Stuttgart 1983.

Jores, Arthur: *Die Medizin in der Krise unserer Zeit,* Bern—Stuttgart 1961.

Marquardt, Hanne: *Reflex Zone Therapy of the Feet,* Thorsons, Wellingborough 1983.

Porkert, Manfred: *The Theoretical Foundations of Chinese Medicine,* Cambridge, Mass. 1974.

St Pierre, Gaston and Boater, Debbie: *The Metamorphic Technique,* Element Books, London 1982.

Wagner, Franz: *Medizin zwischen Utopie und Wissenschaft,* Linz 1984.

Wagner, Franz: *Akupressur Leicht gemacht,* Munich 1985.

Wagner, Franz: *Reflexzonenmassage für jeden,* Munich 1987.

Wagner, Franz: *Medizin im Spannungsfeld von Leiblichkeit und Sozialität,* Linc 1987.

Zeller, Alfred P.: *Die natürliche Hausapotheke,* Oldenburg 1982.

Index